The One-Eyed Surgeon with Only One Thumb

The One-Eyed Surgeon with Only One Thumb

Adventures with My Dad, Harry C. Barber, MD, FACS

John C Barber, MD, FAAO

Copyright © 2017 by John C Barber, MD, FAAO.

Library of Congress Control Number: 2017911589
ISBN: Hardcover 978-1-5434-3914-4
Softcover 978-1-5434-3913-7
eBook 978-1-5434-3912-0

All rights reserved. No part of this book may be reproduced or transmitted in any form or by any means, electronic or mechanical, including photocopying, recording, or by any information storage and retrieval system, without permission in writing from the copyright owner.

Any people depicted in stock imagery provided by Thinkstock are models, and such images are being used for illustrative purposes only.
Certain stock imagery © Thinkstock.

Print information available on the last page.

Rev. date: 07/26/2017

To order additional copies of this book, contact:
Xlibris
1-888-795-4274
www.Xlibris.com
Orders@Xlibris.com
762449

In memory of my father, Harry C. Barber, MD, FACS,
my mentor and inspiration

HARRY CLAY BARBER CAME FROM the humble background of a farm boy in rural Missouri. Through exceptionally hard work, intelligence, and tenacity, he overcame poverty and a teenage hunting injury to become a physician and surgeon and a local leader in the health care of a midsized town in Illinois. He had a tremendous influence on the doctors around him. His character and dedication were powerful inspirations to his fellow physicians and to me as I practiced medicine.

His humility and empathy with patients guided my practice and my interaction with patients. His practice was marked by morality and integrity. He never forgot his humble background, and his warm nature made him a man with many friends.

Chapter 1

Harry was born on January 20, 1904, in a log cabin on a farm near the small town of Orrick, Missouri, which is a few miles from the Ray County seat of Richmond, Missouri. Orrick is a river town about twenty miles downstream from Kansas City. The family farm overlooked the bottom land of the Missouri River from a bluff north of the river.

Harry's family had a rich history of independent pioneering people who migrated from Europe to Virginia and the Carolinas and then moved across the country to push the frontier as it moved to Kentucky and then to Missouri.

My father told me that when the California gold rush occurred in 1849, his grandfather, Travers McCarty Barber, drove a herd of about one hundred mules from Kentucky to California to sell them to the prospectors. He made enough money from that endeavor to return from California by clipper ship around South America to New Orleans. He traveled up the Mississippi and the Missouri Rivers by riverboat to Orrick, Missouri, where he homesteaded a quarter section of land for a farm. He returned to Kentucky to live near his parents until they died. Then he moved, with his wife and children, to establish the farm in Missouri.

My father also told me that he thought we were descendants of Stonewall Jackson. My grandfather Barber's middle name was Gaines, and there was also a woman named Jackson who married a man with the last name of Baber (correct spelling, grandmother's side), several generations before my dad.

However, when I read a biography of Stonewall Jackson, I learned that Stonewall only had one child, a daughter, who never married and did not have children. Stonewall did spend several years as a young boy in Gaines Mills, Virginia, living with a Gaines family, who were in some way related to him, so there may be some connection.

I have a typewritten bound book that my father gave me that was written by John R. Martin, titled *Valentine Martin of Cumberland County Virginia*. It traces the family from Martin Martin and Sarah Hix, the parents of Valentine Martin, through the generations until my generation. My father's lineage, on his mother's side, is traced in that book.

Reading through the book, I learned a lot about Dad's ancestors and why he inherited the strength and determination to rise from a country farm boy to a respected physician and surgeon and prominent member of the community.

From this book, I learned that his great-great-great-great-grandfather, on his mother's side, had lived in Virginia. It traced his family on his mother's side back to Huguenot settlers who came to America as the earliest settlers of Southern Virginia, escaping religious persecution by Catholics in France. Several of his ancestors were ministers; most were in the "Hard Shell" branch of the Baptist Church.

My father's earliest ancestor that John R. Martin could trace was probably named Martin Martin six generations back. He lived in Goochland County, Virginia, which is now called Cumberland County. One of his sons was Valentine Martin who married Jane Bridgewater. They had eleven children. Valentine lived on a stream in Goochland County, Virginia, called Cat Tail Branch. Cat Tail Branch flowed into the Willis River, not far from Gaines Mills.

When Valentine died, he left a large section of land that he divided between his male children.

Land and livestock were the two things of much value to the farmers in southern Virginia. This is illustrated by the will of Valentine Martin that is in John Martin's book and reads as follows (errors included):

> In the name of God, Amen. May The 21, 1758 I, Valentine Martin, being sick and weak but in perfect senses, mind and memory, doth make this my last Will and Testament in manner and form as followth, Viz:
>
> Item. I give and bequeath to my son Orson Martain, two hundred acres of land and plantation whereon he now dwells, to him and his heirs forever. I give and bequeath to my son Orson Martain, six head of cattle to him and his heirs forever.
>
> Item. I give and bequeath to my son Valentine Martain, one hundred acres of land joining Orson's land, to him and his heirs forever.
>
> Item. I give and bequeath to my son Jcbe Martain, one hundred acres of land, to him and his heirs forever. The land joining to Valentine's land.
>
> Item. I give and bequeath to my two sons, that is, Samuel and Isom, The land whereon I now dwell to be equally divided between them. Isom having the plantation on his part, but if Isom should die without an heir, my will and desire is that my son John Martain may have his part of the land.

Item. I give and bequeath to my son John Martain, one shilling Stearlin.

Item. I give and bequeath to my daughter Ester Bond, one shilling Stearlin.

Item. I give and bequeath to my daughter, Sarah Cunningham, one cow and calf. I give and bequeath to my daughter Jane Boatwright, one cow and calf. I give and bequeath to my daughter Mildred, one cow and calf and one bed of new feathers, and furniture. I give and bequeath to my daughter Ann Martain, one featherbed and furniture and a cow and calf.

Item. I give and bequeath the remainder part of my estate to my beloved wife, to do as she shall think proper. My desire is that my estate be not appraised. I nominate and appoint my beloved wife, executrix of this my last will and testament.

      (signed)   (his mark)
      Valentine Martain

Names of witnesses:
Sam Taylor
David Thompson
Samuel Bridgewater.

There is no explanation for the change in spelling for the last name from Martin to Martain (except, possibly, the later Anglicizing of the French Huguenot name). Apparently son John and daughter

Ester were disinherited by the bequest of "one shilling stearlin." Otherwise, the sons inherited land and houses while the daughters received featherbeds and/or a cow and calf. Valentine's son Orson Martin Sr. followed the same pattern with his will.

A son of Valentine Martin, John Martin was with Daniel Boone in Kentucky in 1775 and probably earlier. He served in the Revolutionary War.

Many of my father's ancestors fought in the civil war, mostly for the South. Abner Martin and two of his sons fought for the confederacy. Benjamin Rush Martin also fought for the confederacy and died at the Battle of Malvern Hill near Richmond. Abner and his son, Joseph Addison Martin, fought in the Battle of Five Forks.

The book identifies the battle as the Battle of Five Oaks, but states it was one of Lee's last battles. That would make it the battle now called the Battle of Five Forks near Dinwiddie Courthouse, which is close to Petersburg, Virginia. One skirmish of that battle is known as the Battle of Fair Oaks. Both Abner and Joseph survived the battle to return home where they both died of cholera five weeks after the battle. Other relatives survived various battles, married, and had many children.

One of Dad's ancestors had a son named Madison Hampton, who died before the age of one year. The next child was a son whom they named Second Madison Hampton. He survived and went by the name "Sec." This was on my grandmother's side.

One of John Martin's daughters, Hannah Martin, married Obadiah Baber in 1782. Obadiah and his two brothers, Stanley and Elisha, came to Virginia from Ireland. A few years after the marriage, they moved to Clark County, Kentucky. One of Obadiah's sons, Thomas Baber, married Clarissa Gordon (a Scotch lass) in 1829. Thomas rode on horseback to Ray County, Missouri, where he purchased 640 acres of land for $1.25 per acre ($800.00 total) near

Richmond, Virginia. He returned to Kentucky until 1836 when he brought his family to Missouri by covered wagon. He set the family pattern of working by night and going to school during the day to further his education. When he was nineteen, he got a job on a flatboat that carried tobacco from Ohio to New Orleans. He obtained a business partner and carried cargo on the Ohio and Mississippi Rivers. He eventually became captain of a riverboat that went from Cincinnati to New Orleans. He is known in some references as Squire Baber, the man who built the house on the 640 acres.

Thomas Baber was the father of Benjamin Franklin Baber, my father's grandfather. Benjamin fought in the Confederate Army and survived to marry Margaret Magill. They had ten children. One son, John Franklin Baber, who was my father's uncle, went to Washington University in St. Louis and became a dentist and a leader in the Missouri chapter of the Knights Templar. A daughter, Sarah Mable Baber (known to my father as Aunt Sally), married Young Drayton Craven who was the medical doctor who was the inspiration to his nephew Harry Barber, my father. John and Sarah's sister Myrtle Matilda Baber married Harvey Gaines Barber. I remember my father reciting a poem that says, "Change the name, but not the letter, Change for the worse and not for the better." They were married for many years and had five children, including Harry Clay Barber. Harry was named after two of his uncles, Harry Carr Baber and Edwin Clay Baber.

My grandfather, Harvey Gaines Barber, told the author of the Valentine Martin book that he had an immigrant ancestor, probably Scottish, who entered the country at Charleston, South Carolina, before the Revolutionary War. This was oral history, and Harvey could not trace his family from that ancestor.

The John Martin book picks up the Barber family with my great-grandfather, Travers McCarty Barber. It was his son, Harvey Gaines

Barber, who married Myrtle Matilda Baber, daughter of Benjamin Franklin Baber

Myrtle was born in a big two-story brick house on a large farm near Richmond, Missouri. When I visited that house with my father in the 1950s, it belonged to the editor of the Richmond, Missouri, newspaper. The foundation had settled, causing the floors to be uneven, so the doors were cut at angles to fit the shifted doorjambs. My father showed me where the slave quarters had been torn down behind the house. The well was still there where the Babers had hidden the slaves from the Kansas raiders and local abolitionists who rode through Missouri trying to free slaves. Dad told me that the slaves were lowered down into the well and stood on a brick shelf, just above water level where butter, milk, and other perishables were stored next to the cool water. After the raiders had left, they raised the slaves from the well with the rope and crank used to lift water buckets.

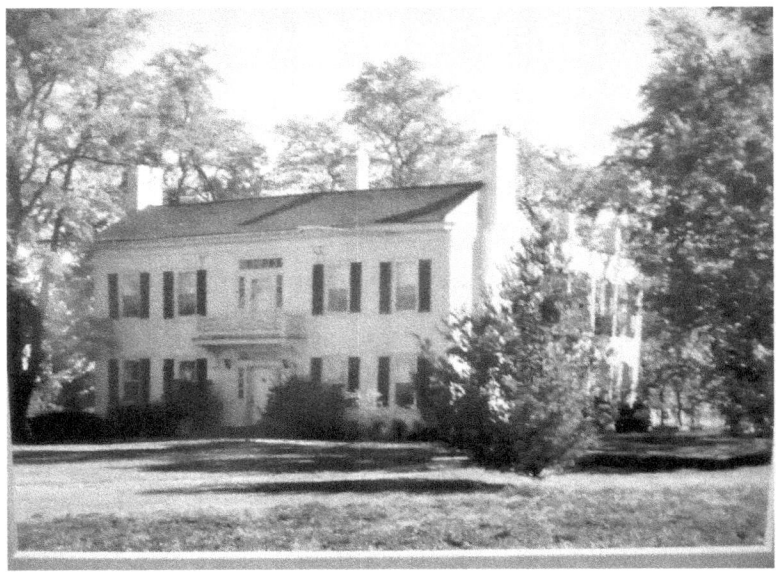

House built by Squire Baber in 1851-54. Squire Baber was Harry Barber's great-great Grandfather.

The house was built by Squire Baber in 1851–54. A story related in the book *Ray County, 1973*, tells of local secret abolitionist raiders trying to capture one of Squire's five sons who served in the Confederate army. After promising to retrieve his son who was sleeping upstairs, Squire retreated to the second floor where he and his sons fired on the raiders from several windows to make it look like there were many men in the house. One disguised raider who happened to be from Richmond was hit in the foot, causing him to lose his anonymity, forcing him to leave Richmond.

Several miles away and years later, my father was one of five children on a farm near Orrick, Missouri. He told me that he and his brothers Frank, Olin, and Charlie and a sister, Ruth, slept in a loft above the one-room cabin. They were typical farmers who lived off the land. They raised garden crops and canned them for the winter, and they kept chickens, hogs, and cows. Plowing and some other chores were done with the aid of their one horse.

Dad told me that the children rode the horse or walked to a one-room school and carried a hot baked potato in their pockets as a hand warmer on cold winter mornings. When they got to school, they put their potato on the stove that heated the schoolroom to keep it warm until lunchtime when they ate the potato. They put rocks on the stove after lunch to use as hand warmers on the way home. One of the problems of going to school was adapting to wearing shoes, which were uncomfortable after going barefoot all summer.

After finishing everything that was taught in the one-room country school, Dad went to high school in Richmond. Boys of high school age who lived on farms were needed for farm work in the spring and fall, so he could not attend school until after the crops were harvested in the fall and then only until plowing and planting time began in the spring. My father was so hungry for an education that he read the entire textbook for each course, so he did not miss much by being out of school for farm work.

His father realized that he was smart, so he wanted him to graduate from high school. One of the main requirements for graduating from high school was completion of one year of algebra. By the end of his third year, my father had not taken algebra because of starting school late and finishing early every year. His father allowed him to go to school and skip farm work, except for weekends, the whole school year for his senior year so that he could take algebra and graduate. He graduated from high school in about 1920.

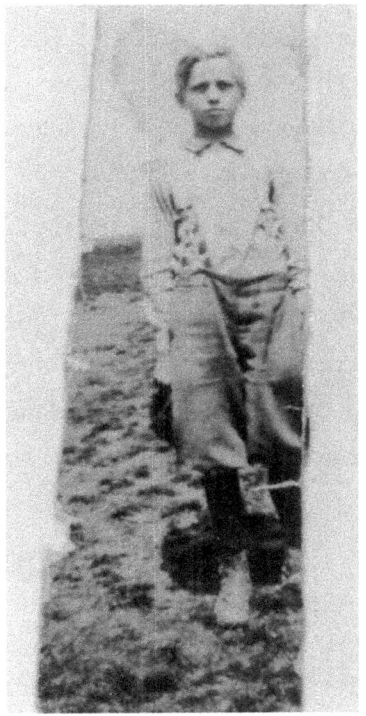

Harry C. Barber on the last day of school, about 1917.

Living on the farm, my father developed a passion for hunting. He hunted rabbits and other varmints for food, but his real enthusiasm was for shooting waterfowl along the nearby Missouri River. The farm was on top of a hill above the river bottoms. Every fall, when he could get away from the farm work, he would walk a mile down to the river with his shotgun to shoot ducks and geese to help feed the family.

He would roam up and down the river looking for birds to shoot. One day, when he was seventeen, he put his shotgun down over a fence before climbing the fence. He said it was an inexpensive mail-order shotgun from Sears. In retrospect, he was certain that the safety was on, but the gun fired accidentally and shot off his left thumb. When the surgeon was finished removing the mangled thumb, there was a star-shaped scar where the thumb had been. That scar would move and dimple slightly when he tried to move the absent thumb. When he wanted to hold something with his left hand, he would wrap his fingers around the object. He developed a strong grip with the fingers of his left hand.

One pellet from the shotgun went into his left eye and caused an infection. There were no antibiotics then in about 1920, so the infection made it necessary to remove his eye before the infection could spread to his brain. (Sulfa, the first true antibiotic, was first used in about 1935. Penicillin was not widely used clinically until about 1941.)

After he lost his eye, he wore a glass eye that matched his other eye very well. I did not know that his left eye was artificial until I was in high school. Most of his patients did not know that he could only see with one eye.

While he was in medical school, he was introduced to a young ocularist, Fritz Reinhart, who was from Germany. Fritz had been taught to make glass artificial eyes, in Germany, by his father. He was a glass artist who made his own glass and shaped it into shells that fit on the blind eyeball or prosthesis under the eyelids. He colored the glass to look like the iris and sclera of the good eye and used pigment dust and red glass rods, heated and drawn thin to make vessels to change the background color of the white part of the artificial eye to match the good eye of his patient.

Dad told me that every two years, the artificial eye would start to feel rough and his eye would start to make excessive mucous. Dad would have to get a new glass eye. He tried the prosthetic eyes made from plastic, but they became rough and irritating almost immediately. He was probably having giant papillary conjunctivitis from the plastic eye like modern contact lens wearers experience today. By the time he started his practice, he would go to St. Louis every other year to see Fritz to get a new eye. Fritz would polish the old eye in his kiln to make it a usable backup should anything happen to the new eye.

When Dad was about seventy years old, Fritz tried to retire to live in Colorado. The people who knew how to make glass artificial eyes were a dying breed. While I was practicing ophthalmology, I tried to find someone who could make Dad his glass eyes, but I could not find an oculist who would work in glass. Dad and Fritz's other patients put enough pressure on him to convince him to come out of retirement for two months every summer to service his old customers. He would make enough glass every winter in his basement glass furnace to supply his own glass for the eyes.

Dad said that having only one eye made him a better shot with a shotgun. He shot right-handed, so he lined his right eye with the gun barrel and pointed it at or ahead of the bird and pulled the trigger.

Later, when I would go quail hunting with him, he almost always had two birds dead on the ground while I was still trying to pick a bird in the covey to shoot. When the covey flushed, he would look for two birds close together to shoot with his first shot and then look for a third before they flew out of range.

He taught me how to fire a rifle and a shotgun and the basics of gun safety before I was twelve years old. I could never equal his marksmanship with either a rifle or shotgun.

Dad took my brother and me out into the country to shoot tin cans with the rifle. The cans were lined up in front of a creek bank for a backstop. Dad taught us how to hunt rabbits and squirrels with a .22 rifle and pheasants and ducks with shotguns. He also taught us how to clean and dress the animals and birds, so anything we shot, we had to dress and eat. My mother was very good at cooking wild game, but she refused to dress what we shot.

CHAPTER 2

AFTER GRADUATING FROM HIGH SCHOOL, Harry enrolled for the summer in the Southwest Missouri State Teachers College, formerly the Fourth District Normal School, in Springfield, Missouri. He obtained a teacher's certificate that summer so that he could return home to teach in a country school. He taught in two different one-room schools during the next three years while living at home to save his money.

He took me to see the little one-room Enterprise School, where he taught thirty-six pupils from first through the eighth grades in 1922–23. In a note he made in his copy of *Ray County, 1978*, he wrote that "the school was originally known as the J.L. Sullivan School. The school and nearby church were built and donated by Mr. Sullivan to the community of early settlers." The community later became known as Enterprise. We drove around in the area, but he could not find his other school, the Fitch School. We later learned from the locals that it had been torn down several years before.

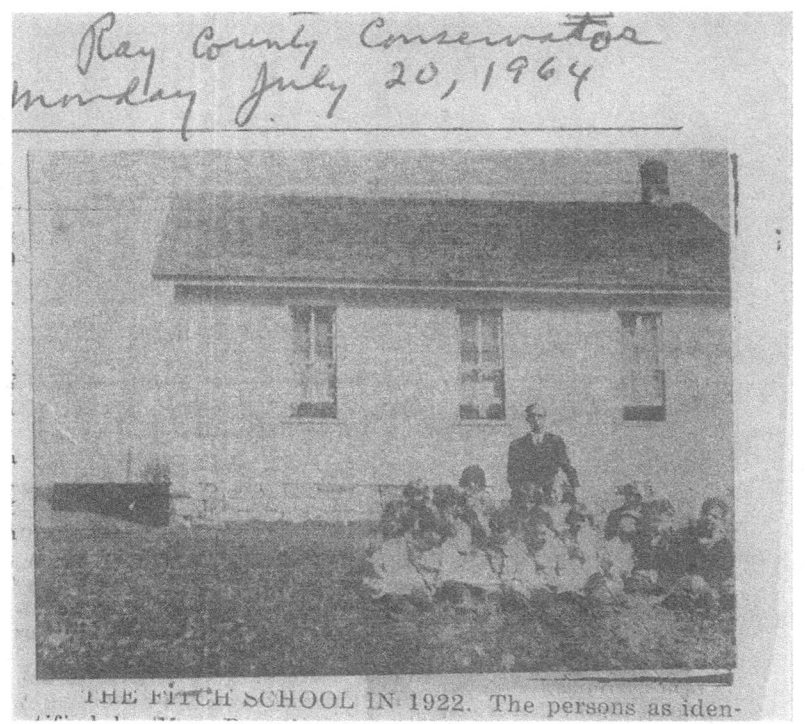

Clipping from the Ray County Conservator of July 20, 1964 showing Harry Barber with his students at the Fitch School in 1922.

His family had built a larger farmhouse by the time he finished high school, so he was not living in the loft. Living at home those three years allowed him to save enough money to enroll at the University of Missouri in Columbia, Missouri.

His goal was to become a doctor like his uncle Young, so he majored in biology. When I asked him why he became a doctor and whether it was because of his injury, he told me that he always wanted to become a doctor and was not deterred by the loss of his left thumb and his decreased depth perception from the loss of his left eye. He explained that after several years, he regained some depth perception.

He got a job reading electric meters, which he did after classes and on weekends. He told me that he would wait until Saturday afternoon during the football game to read the meter at the stadium. His meter book and flashlight would gain him admission to the stadium without a ticket. Once he had read the meter, he stayed for the game. I am not sure that it was time to read the meter every time there was a home game, but the gatekeepers did not know when the meter was due to be read. Dad always had a way with people that helped him do a lot of things.

He told me about being present for the first game in the new stadium that had been completed just weeks before the first game of the football season. He said that it had rained for a week before the game and the field had not had a chance to grow grass, so it was a sea of mud. The kickoff was high and came down pointed to the ground. The ball stuck, half buried in the mud. He described the game as a total mud bath for both teams. When he told me about that game, he could not remember who won.

After high school and three years of teaching, he was over twenty-one and had become a Master Mason in the Richmond Lodge. Many college students during that era had worked for several years before deciding to attend college, so they were older than the average student of today. He joined the Acacia Fraternity and lived in the fraternity house. At that time, only Master Masons could belong to Acacia. As students became younger, the fraternity rule was relaxed to require being recommended by two Masons. Acacia fraternity still has strong ties to the Masonic orders.

When he was an active member of the fraternity, the actives quizzed the pledges about the university. There are six tall columns in the middle of campus that are all that is left of Academic Hall after it was destroyed by fire. One of the favorite questions was to tell the pledges that the columns were not all the same distance apart. The pledges were to find out which two columns were farthest apart. The pledges would go the columns and measure the distance between them very carefully. When they returned with the data and the conclusion of which two were the farthest apart by their measurements, the actives would tell the pledges that they were wrong and send them back to measure again. The answer they were looking for was that the two columns that were farthest apart were the columns at either end of the row. I do not know if hazing got any worse than that in the 1920s, but it probably did.

During the summer months, Dad sold aluminum ware, door-to-door, to raise money for school. That ended when someone stole his aluminum products sample case from the fraternity house. He had left it in the foyer, where everyone hung their coats, when it disappeared. He never found the case or discovered who took it.

When school was in session, he waited tables at a women's boardinghouse to finance his schooling. He worked his way through college and obtained both bachelor of arts and bachelor of science degrees.

He also had a job working in the chemistry laboratories. On his shift, he was in charge of "the cage"—the locked room where chemicals, glassware, and other materials were issued. This was during Prohibition, so the absolute ethanol that was essential for certain chemical reactions was kept there under lock and key. There was a logbook to keep track of the ethanol as it was dispensed. They had to report how much was dispensed, by whom, to whom, and record any spillage each time they dispensed the alcohol so they could account for all of the alcohol.

Dad learned that they allowed 5 cc of spillage for every time alcohol was dispensed. The cage workers usually did not spill any alcohol, but faithfully recorded 5 cc of spillage for every pour. At the end of the month, the laboratory workers had a party to consume the "spilled" ethanol.

This was at odds with what my father told me about alcohol when I was growing up. He told me that he had an uncle and a brother who had become alcoholics years after his college days. It was known by the time he gave me this advice that alcohol dependency ran in families. He told me that he never drank because he was afraid that he might like it too much and become an alcoholic. He advised me not to drink alcohol because our family had the alcoholism gene. When I was growing up, my father never drank because he was on call twenty-four hours a day, seven days a week, fifty-two weeks a year. I learned that throughout the time he practiced medicine, he would have one highball each year and that only on New Year's Eve at a party with friends.

After he retired and moved to Arkansas, he would have one highball before dinner—Old Grand-Dad with 7Up. My mother would have a glass of New York State Catawba grape wine along with him.

Once, when we were in St. Thomas, Virgin Islands, on a Christmas vacation, my brother, Bruce, who was in college then, ordered a second drink during dinner as Bluebeard's Castle. He made the comment that he "could not fly on one wing." My father launched into a lecture on the dangers of drinking to excess, like having a second drink. My mother immediately ordered a second "Bluebeard's Wench," a potent rum drink of the house. The evening rapidly went downhill from there.

Dad's undergraduate grades were good enough to get him into the two-year basic science medical school a Missouri U in Columbia. He had an uncle, in Richmond, John Baber, the dentist. The uncle had taken anatomy of the head as part of his training at Washington University Dental School. He told my father that he should have a skull to study so that he could learn all the anatomical details of the skull. There are many holes in the skull for nerves and blood vessels and depressions or ridges for attachment of muscles, etc.

In those days, some of the medical schools had freshman students acquire their own cadaver to dissect in the anatomy course. Some students bought bodies from poor families who could not afford burials. Others hired "resurrection men" to steal bodies from graves. Fortunately, Missouri U Medical School supplied enough cadavers so that he did not have to bring his own.

His uncle John was also the coroner for Ray County, Missouri. One day, he appeared at my father's house with a heavy bag. When my father opened the bag, he found a human head from which all the skin and most of the muscles had been removed. His uncle told him to boil it in lye to remove the remaining tissues and to saw off the top on the skull with a hack saw to remove the brains. Once the top of the skull was removed, the internal ridges and holes could be seen.

When my father asked his uncle where the skull came from, he replied that there was a black man, who was a pauper and whose family could not afford burial fees, who was now buried in a somewhat shortened coffin, courtesy of the county.

My father told me that he boiled the head too long and made some of the thin bones brittle. He was able to remove all the tissues from the bones to make a good skull for studying. He took the skull to medical school and used it to study. He inserted pipe cleaners into the various holes from the outside to determine where each hole came out on the inside to track nerves and blood vessels. When I started medical school, he gave the skull to me to help me learn anatomy. I still have it.

While he was in medical school, he continued to wait tables at the boardinghouse for women students. That is where he met Edith, my mother. He was very taken by Edith's looks and manners, so he asked her to the fraternity's Valentine's Day dance. They continued to date through his medical school years. My mother was from a prominent St. Louis family, but she was attracted to this poor, but intelligent farm boy who waited tables.

After his first year of medical school, my father managed to get a job on a crew that was laying a pipeline across Missouri. There was a big machine that dug the trench for the pipe, but when the machine hit clay or rock, the men had to get down in the ditch and dig with picks, shovels, and occasional dynamite.

At the end of his first day on the job, Dad's hands were covered with blisters. He asked the foreman if there was something that would help his blisters. The foreman asked him why his hands were so soft and white. My father told him that he had been studying in the anatomy laboratory at medical school and the formaldehyde in the cadavers had made his hands soft. The foreman told Dad that he was looking for someone smart enough to carry the dynamite, and he thought that a medical student must be smart. He asked my father to carry the dynamite rather than dig the ditch.

My father was smart. The first thing he did was to take the box of blasting caps out of the dynamite box to make it less dangerous. This meant that he had to make two trips every time he had to move the dynamite. He told me that about two days after he started carrying the dynamite, he stumbled and dropped the dynamite box. Since the blasting caps were not in the box, nothing happened. After that, he did not mind taking two trips to move the dynamite.

Between his second and third years of medical school, he worked at the state mental hospital in Fulton, Missouri. Fulton State Hospital was opened in 1851 and was the oldest mental health hospital west of the Mississippi River.

He worked as a technician who drew blood samples from patients and then prepared slides for the pathologists to examine for evidence of malaria. The first thing he did was to construct a wooden box to organize the tubes of blood and the syringes, needles, and other paraphernalia for drawing blood. Hospital blood technicians today use a similar box when they go from room to room to draw blood.

When he explained this search for malaria, he told me that advanced, or tertiary, syphilis affected the brain and caused mental illness. Many of the patients in the mental hospital were there because of syphilis affecting their brains. Penicillin had not been discovered, so there was no good drug for neurosyphilis. Heavy metal shots of arsenic, bismuth, and mercury salts, given in painful deep hip injections, were used for primary and secondary syphilis, but they did not work for tertiary or neurosyphilis.

The popular way to treat neurosyphilis at that time was to induce high fevers because *Treponema pallidum*, the spirochete organism that causes syphilis, could not tolerate temperatures much above normal body temperature of 98.6°F. The doctors injected malaria organisms into the patients to give them the high fevers of malaria (104°F to 106°F). These fevers occurred from every other day to every four days, or longer, depending on the type of malaria. The doctors allowed the fevers to continue until they thought the treponema of syphilis were dead from the high body temperatures. Then the patients were treated for malaria, usually with quinine or Atabrine (quinacrine).

The patient's blood smears were examined every few days after treatment of the malaria to see if the malaria parasites were still present in the bloodstream, indicating that the patient needed further treatment. The malaria organism is a parasite that lives in the red blood cells of its victim. There are now five known types of malaria, but they used the three types that were known at that time. Each type has three distinctive stages of development in the red blood cells, so each type of malaria required several slides to demonstrate the stages of the disease.

My father knew that the set of teaching microscopic slides that was supplied to each student at the Missouri U Medical School did not have good slides for malaria. Since the slides at the hospital were discarded after they were read, he saved many sets of slides showing the various stages of the disease for the three types of malaria. He presented the slides that he had collected and labeled to the Missouri U Pathology Department at the end of that summer.

In the 1920s, at the end of the two years of basic science medical school, the students at Missouri University had to transfer to a clinical medical school in which to take the last two years of clinical training for a medical degree. Washington University, in St. Louis, accepted Dad into the medical class for the last two years.

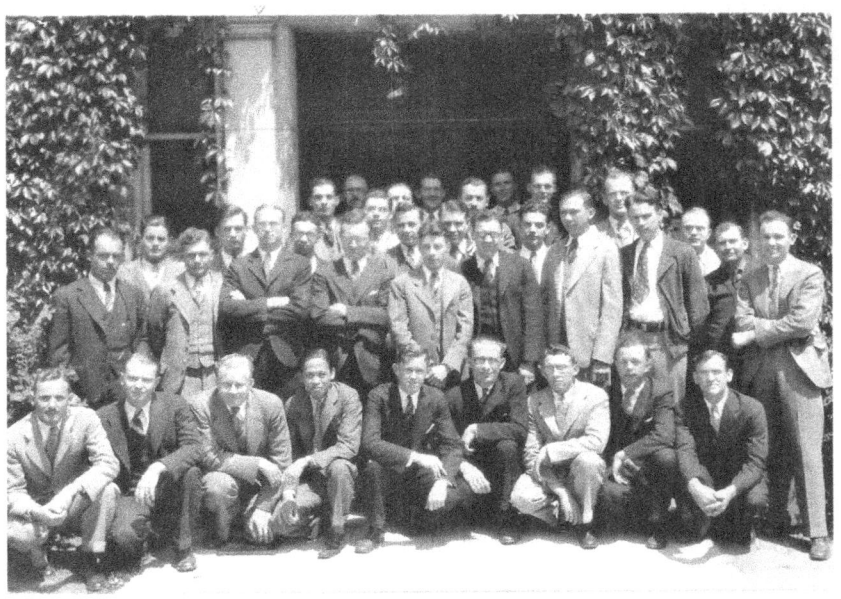

Photograph of the Second Year Class of
University of Missouri Medical School, Spring,
1927 Harry Barber is third from left in first
row of standing students. (Arms crossed)

My father had another uncle, who was a physician, Dr. Young D. Cravens. Uncle Young died while my father was in the first year of medical school at Missouri U. He left his wife, Aunt Sally Cravens, the house, his car, and a significant amount of money. Since Uncle Young had been a mentor to my dad, Sally decided to use some of her money to help my father through medical school so he could follow her husband's footsteps. Aunt Sally paid his tuition and gave him some money to allow him to live in the Phi Beta Pi medical fraternity house about three blocks from the Washington University medical school. It was much less expensive than living in an apartment.

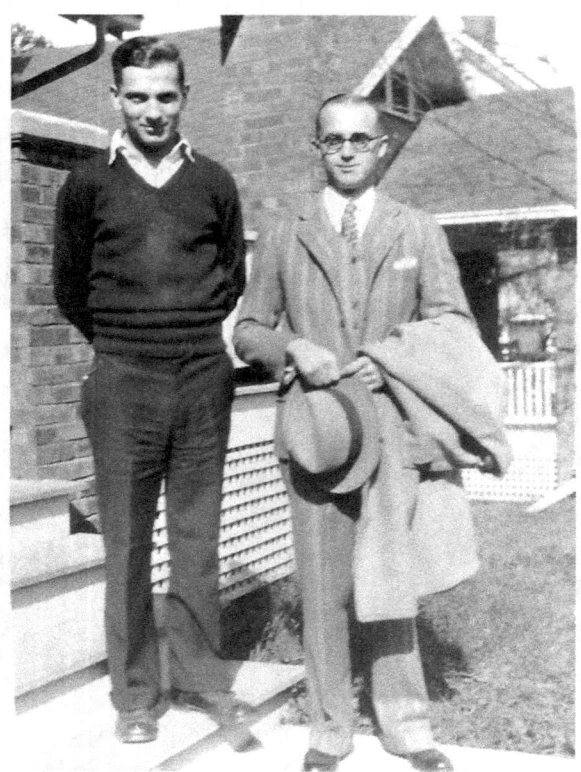

Harry Barber (with hat and coat) with his cousin Forrest Baber at Washington University School of Medicine, 1929.

The clinical years were too demanding to allow him to work part-time during school. The clinical years were in session continuously except for a short summer break. Aunt Sally continued to help him with money for school and to help pay his room and board. When he started medical school in St. Louis, he needed transportation for himself and his belongings. Aunt Sally had Uncle Young's automobile that she could not drive, so she allowed my father to drive it to St. Louis, park it there, and then drive it home when he returned. He was not to drive it anywhere else. No joy riding!

Dad was still dating Edith when she was home in St. Louis. One beautiful spring day, he offered to drive her through Forrest Park, which was across King's Highway from the medical school. His cousin, Forrest Baber, also a medical student, saw them and wasted no time in reporting the infraction to Aunt Sally. When my father returned to Richmond at the end of his third medical year, Sally took the car away and told him there would be no more tuition money either because he had broken the rules.

My father was devastated. He had one more year of medical school before he could graduate, but no tuition money. He had received a loan from the Indiana branch of the Knights Templar to partially pay for his living expenses but it was not enough to pay his tuition. No doubt that this loan was through the influence of his uncle John, who was an officer in the Knights Templar in Missouri.

Dad told Edith about his situation, and she told her father. Her father knew my father by this time and was impressed by his desire to become a doctor. He gave money to Edith to loan to my father so that he could finish medical school. I learned when I read my father's letters after he died that he had signed notes to my mother to repay the money. The letters mentioned that he had paid some of the notes off, but I think there were still some unpaid notes when they married and made the payback moot.

My father told many stories about life in the Phi Beta House. Tom Bricker was a medical student who lived on the top floor of the house. Most evenings, about ten o'clock, everyone would hear loud banging noises coming from his room. Both Tom and his roommate would take a study break and wrestle in their room for ten to twenty minutes. No one else in the house could study because of the noise.

I worked with Dr. Bricker when I was in my internship. He was one of the best surgeons I ever watched or assisted, and there were many good surgeons at Washington University Medical School. I learned that Dr. Bricker managed to work a game of handball or tennis into his schedule almost every day. He remembered my father, but did not tell me any stories about him.

Dad's medical school years were during Prohibition, so some of the students made ginger beer and bathtub gin at the Phi Beta House. They would hide the beer in the back of the closets under their clothes. Some of the bottles would explode in the closet as the beer fermented and aged. This had a fragrant effect on the clothes in the closet.

About the time that my father graduated from medical school, in 1930, my mother-to-be broke up with him and started dating a guy named Richard. (I never learned his last name.) My father started his internship at Missouri Baptist Hospital in St. Louis. He was on duty in the hospital every other night and every other weekend, so he was too busy to date anyone seriously. He told me that he earned $25 a month, lived in the hospital, and was furnished all meals and uniforms. The interns all "borrowed" soap and toothpaste from the ward supplies to save money.

His search for a job started near the end of his rotating internship. A rotating internship has periods on internal medicine, obstetrics/gynecology, pediatrics, and surgical services rather than only one service. He could not afford to continue into residency training in a specialty, but he could get a license to practice general medicine after completing the rotating internship. He learned about an opening as the assistant physician in a small-town practice in Normal, Illinois. He applied for the job and was hired.

My father told me that he was offered an expenses-paid residency position at the new Malcolm Bliss Hospital in St. Louis if he would do a residency in psychiatry. Malcolm Bliss was a large mental hospital near downtown St. Louis. It was the hospital where the mentally ill and criminally ill patients were hospitalized. There was also a large population of "recovering" alcoholics. The image of that hospital did not appeal to my father, so he took the general practice position in Normal.

When his internship ended in June, he immediately moved to Normal and started assisting Dr. Ferdinand McCormick in his office. In those days, most family doctors did everything in medicine—heart attacks, high blood pressure, diabetes, uncomplicated surgery, delivering babies, setting fractures, easing the pain of the dying, even diagnosing psychiatric illness—everything.

As he worked with Dr. McCormick, he did all the weekend call, night call, and surgical assisting in addition to seeing his half of the office patients. He claimed that he was paid $150 per month and was glad to have a job during the Depression.

Several weeks after he started to practice in Normal, he learned that blood transfusions were still being done by the push-pull method. The donor and recipient were lined up side by side on gurneys. A needle, connected to a tube, was put in a vein in each patient. The two tubes were joined at a stopcock connected to a large syringe. The stopcock was turned to connect the syringe with the donor, and blood was drawn into the syringe. The stopcock was turned to connect with the recipient, and the blood was injected from the syringe into their vein. This was repeated until the desired amount had been transfused. The procedure had to be done rapidly before the blood could clot and block the tubing. However, drawing and injecting blood too fast could damage the red blood cells and release potassium from the cells, causing a toxic level of potassium in the blood of the recipient.

During his internship, my father had learned to do transfusions using citrate in the blood. In this procedure, a measured amount of sterile citrate is put in the sterile flask that was used to collect blood from the donor. The flask is swirled during collection to mix the citrate with the blood as it enters the flask to keep the blood from clotting. The flask containing the blood mixed with citrate is then taken to the recipient patient's room where it was hung to deliver the blood intravenously by gravity. In those days, citrated blood could be kept in a refrigerator for several hours until it is used. The donor and recipient did not have to be in the same room.

My father did the first citrated blood transfusion in Bloomington–Normal. He announced that he was going to do it and drew an audience of several nurses and doctors. The hospital soon adopted this method of blood transfusion.

During that first year of practice, my father received a letter from my mother saying that Richard had not turned out to be the love of her life and she still loved my father and wanted him to take her back. Dad answered the letter saying that he did not have time to keep a wife happy and would have to place the welfare of his patients above home life. I have the letter in which my mother says she loved him very much and she could be happy just keeping my father happy if he would only take her back. She convinced him that she could make life easier for him to care for his patients and promised to never complain that she was neglected because of his patients.

When he received that letter, he was still in love with her and gladly took her back. The engagement was announced in the St. Louis and Normal papers on November 30, 1933. On February 10, 1934, they were married in the Union Avenue Christian Church in St. Louis, near her parents' house on Pershing Avenue in the DeBaliviere District, near Forest Park.

I did not know until I was in high school that Mom had been raised by Christian Scientist parents and that she gave up that religion when she married my father. She remained very distrustful of doctors for the rest of her life when her own health was concerned.

After a few years in Dr. McCormick's practice, shortly after they were married, Dr. McCormick told my father that he could become a very good surgeon if he had some surgery training. Dr. McCormick sent my father and mother to Philadelphia for six months and paid their expenses so that Dad could do residency training in general surgery at the University of Pennsylvania Hospital. At that time, full residency training in surgery required three years, but many general practitioners took a year or less of surgical residency training to be able to repair hernias, remove an appendix or tonsils, and do a cesarean section delivery.

When they returned to Normal after his six months of surgical residency, my father assisted Dr. McCormick with surgery and did minor cases himself. Three months after Dad returned, Dr. McCormick, as my father put it, "dropped dead of a heart attack."

Of necessity, my father took over the practice and began doing most kinds of surgery. He had assisted on these types of surgery many times, so it was not much of a jump to be the lead surgeon. He told me that he never electively opened a chest or a skull, but surgery for injuries caused him to explore and close many of them. He was quick to refer anything he thought was beyond his level to appropriate specialists if they were available. At that time, doctors assisted each other at surgery. He usually worked with fully trained surgeons, but soon considered himself as equally capable at doing surgery as they were.

In a letter he wrote to the American College of Surgeons to support his application to that organization, he summarized his surgery from 1936 through 1941 as follows:

Year	1936	1937	1938	1939	1940	1941
Major operations performed:	104	126	120	182	107	151
Assistant surgeon:	196	250	201	260	342	186
Total surgeries	300	276	321	442	509	337

GRAND TOTAL: 2285

(Dad enlisted in the army in 1941. He did very little surgery during his first year in the service while treating young recruits.)

Bloomington–Normal was on one of the first four-lane sections of US Highway 66 that went from Chicago to Los Angeles. There was unlimited access on most of the highway. The other roads crossed US 66 at grade level with two-way stop signs but without stoplights. Many cars turned left onto the first pair of lanes, especially at night, and were going the wrong way, so my father treated many auto accident victims.

Safety glass had not been invented and cars did not have seat belts, so many car collisions resulted in people, especially on the passenger side, going through the windshield. After the collision, sometimes the person who went through the windshield would fall back into the car, going back through the broken windshield, causing many more lacerations.

The drivers were often killed or seriously injured by the steering wheel, because seat belts had not even begun to be installed in cars. Two-door cars with folding bench seats did not have locks on the seatbacks, so backseat passengers were thrown against the seats and pushed the front seat occupants against the dash or through the windshield. Route 66 and US 1 both went through Normal and furnished Dad many patients. The rural speed limit in Illinois was "reasonable and proper," so high speeds were not unusual.

Besides this trauma, his surgery included hernias, gallbladders, appendectomies, hysterectomies, gastric resections, bowel resections, and cancer surgery. He delivered babies until an obstetrics and gynecology doctor moved to town. The same happened with orthopedics and ear, nose, and throat. He saw sore throats, diabetes, hypertension, flu, kidney stones, and diarrhea, basically anything that walked into the office or called for a house call.

One night, he was called out by the police to treat an auto thief who had tried to run a roadblock near Lincoln, Illinois, about thirty miles south of Bloomington–Normal. When the thief had tried to run a roadblock, the state police shot him through the car door with a dumdum shell from a shotgun. (A dumdum shell is a large shotgun shell filled with large shot, about one-fourth-inch size.) The blast had hit him in the stomach. Dad took twenty-three one-fourth-inch pellets out of the man's abdomen and sewed up many holes in his small intestine. Sometimes the pellets had done so much damage that he had to resect a small section of bowel and do an anastomosis of the cut ends. He spent all night, but the patient lived to stand trial.

Chapter 3

My father was greatly influenced by my mother's family. They were prosperous St. Louis Germans. My grandfather grew up on a farm in north St. Louis near the present corner of King's Highway and Natural Bridge Road. My great-grandfather grew vegetables, including white asparagus, to sell to the riverboats that docked in St. Louis. The house was in the middle of a truck farm, but today, it is on Shreve Avenue, a few blocks from Natural Bridge Road. It is surrounded by several two-story houses and many tract houses.

These new houses are all the same externally and run for blocks. My father joked that you could not find your own house if you came home too drunk because they all looked the same. Many had small aluminum awnings of different colors over the front door to distinguish them from the others. Several older houses stood out. My mother told me that her uncles and aunts lived in those houses. She mentioned an Aunt Clara Koester who was different from her aunt Clara "Next Door." Mom's middle name was Clara.

The main house is set back from the street and has an open yard around it. It has two stories plus a dormered attic. It dominated the neighborhood. The architecture bears a striking resemblance to the house in which my grandmother, Myrtle Baber, was born near Richmond, Missouri.

My grandfather did not like farming, so he went into business. He was very successful and invested well, but was caught in the margin crunch on Black Monday, 1929. He lost everything that he had invested when the market crashed. He vowed to make it all back before he died. He eventually became vice president of Carborundum Company and then vice president of Colcord-Wright Machinery & Supply Company. He was a charter member of the Missouri Athletic Club (MAC) and played on their basketball team in interclub competition.

My uncle Roy, Mom's brother, had a stormy career in business and tended to disagree with his bosses, causing him to change jobs a lot. My grandfather bought the Good Taste Cookies Company and was the CEO. He appointed Roy the president of the company to give him a high-paying job with some stability. Roy liked being president of a corporation, but liked the perquisites of the office better than the job. My mother said he spent more time at the University Club and his country club than he did at the office.

One winter night, as my granddad and Roy were leaving the company, they were robbed at gunpoint. My grandfather decided he did not want to be subjected to robbery to make a job for Roy. The next day, Granddad decided to sell the company, so Roy was out of work again. He got a job selling cardboard shipping boxes on the road. He held that job for several years until he quit and started working for a realtor. Good Taste Cookies eventually grew into Archway Cookies, a national brand.

It was customary in St. Louis to publish probate proceedings in the newspaper. These were often the topic of discussions at the Missouri Athletic Club Founders Table where Granddad ate lunch. He told my mother that he hoped that his estate would be reported at more than a million dollars. When he died, his probate report listed his estate at somewhat less than a million dollars plus some rarely traded stock that was not valued. That stock was his holding in Pearl Brewing Company that was still family held. According to my mother, the stock value would have pushed his estate over the million-dollar level, but his friends at the table did not know that.

My grandfather had a brother-in-law, Otto Koehler, who was from Germany and had trained as a brewmaster. My mother told me that Otto had a roving eye and was embarrassing the family, so in the 1880s, my great-grandfather gave him $10,000 to go find and buy a brewery. He went to San Antonio, Texas, to work for Lone Star Brewing. In 1899, he bought the San Antonio Brewing Company out of bankruptcy and became the president of the bankrupt company. He later renamed it Pearl Brewing Company. They started brewing a European-style beer that became very popular, and the brewery was doing very well before Prohibition.

He and Aunt Emma would go back home to Germany every year for a month or more on one of the transatlantic steamships. She would bring back furniture for the mansion they built on top of the hill at 310 West Ashby in San Antonio. From the third floor, Otto could see the brewery several blocks away.

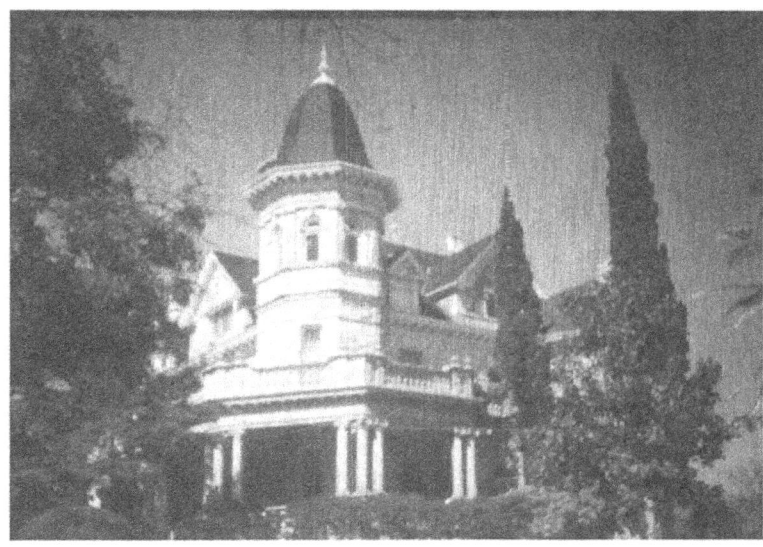

Mansion built by Otto Koehler at 310
West Ashby, San Antonio, Texas.

German workmen were brought over from Germany to do the woodwork, the exterior masonry, and stone carving for the fireplaces. There was an elevator from the basement to the third-floor ballroom because Emma's arthritis was too bad for her to do the stairs. Dad told me that the third floor was a ballroom with a bar along one side. There were etched glass mirrors on the wall behind the bar. My father told me that he considered the etchings to be X-rated. I never saw the ballroom, but I heard that the etched murals had dancing Rubenesque nude women. There was a bar in the basement that always had a fresh keg of Pearl. There was also a bowling alley for the entertainment of their guests. The butler doubled as pin boy.

Uncle Otto and Aunt Emma did not have any children. Of the several years when they went to Germany, they arranged to bring back one of Otto's nieces or nephews. These younger people were brought to the United States as sponsored indentured servants. The two nieces worked as maids in the house. The nephew, who was also named Otto Koehler, worked in the brewery. He eventually went to college and came back to San Antonio to work in the brewery. He worked in management and eventually was named president of the brewery when Emma retired.

My mother told me that in 1914, before Prohibition started, Uncle Otto was shot and killed, for some unknown reason, by either his mistress or the upstairs maid (not one of the nieces), depending on which story you believe. According to an article in the *San Antonio Magazine*, the woman, a prominent woman in San Antonio society, was tried in "one of the most famous murder cases ever tried in Baxer County." She claimed self-defense and was acquitted by a jury in 1918.

After Otto's demise, Tanta Emma stepped in and ran the brewery. She hired a clever manager, Brooks McGimsey, who got the brewery through flooding from the San Antonio River, worker strikes, and low profits during the 1920s and managed to get the brewery through Prohibition.

One of the brewmasters discovered a way to make near beer by killing the fermentation process of Pearl beer before the alcohol reached the legal near-beer level of 0.8 percent. Since it tasted like real beer, it was very popular, but it did not sell the same volume that they had been producing in real beer. Mr. McGimsey decided to use the excess cooling capacity of the beer-cooling equipment to make ice cream to supplement the company sales.

My mother told me that Brooks McGimsey had Koehler family money hidden in many places in case the brewery went bankrupt during the Prohibition. He diversified the company to include ice cream and candy making, dry cleaning, and automobile repairs.

Either because of the diversity or Prohibition, the brewery changed its name to Alamo Industries and then Alamo Foods Company.

The brewery survived and was making near beer, called XXX Pearl, when the Halstead Act (Prohibition) was repealed in 1933. There was a short lapse between the vote to repeal Prohibition and the date when beer could be sold. Since it takes ninety to one hundred days to start up a brewery and produce marketable beer, most of the old breweries were caught flat-footed. They needed to order supplies and tool up before they could make beer.

Pearl had beer fermenting in the tanks to make near beer. They did not kill the fermentation and had full-strength beer in kegs the night Prohibition ended. At midnight, the gates of Pearl opened, and the beer wagons rolled out through the streets of San Antonio with free beer for all. Pearl became the biggest-selling beer in Texas by World War II.

In 1940, Otto Junior (Uncle Otto's nephew) took over the management of the brewery. Emma died in 1943 and left money to over forty-five charitable organizations.

After World War II, Otto could not get along with Brooks McGimsey, who, by this time, owned a significant amount of Pearl stock, so Otto bought out Brooks's Pearl stock. McGimsey used his buyout money and business connections to start the Air Force Bank of San Antonio. This was the bank designated for any member of the US Air Force to direct deposit his paycheck from the service for their family to use while they were stationed anywhere in the world. The bank grew rapidly, so Brooks and his wife, Marietta, did very well. Dad respected Brooks McGimsey's business acumen and often consulted him about stock investments.

Brooks eventually developed cataracts, but refused to have surgery to remove them. He consulted the best ophthalmologists in San

Antonio, and they all advised surgery. He refused surgery because none of these reputable ophthalmologists could ethically guarantee him 20/20 vision after the surgery. His cataracts became hypermature and caused him to develop glaucoma that was hard to control. He went blind from the glaucoma several years before he died, but never had his cataracts removed. Had he gone to an ophthalmologist who unethically guaranteed 20/20 vision after surgery, or if he had been willing to take the risks with his eyes that he took in business, he might have kept his vision.

Brooks was also one of the founders of the San Antonio Country Club. His widow, Marietta McGimsey, insisted that we stop in San Antonio when Letha and I picked up our son Scott from Camp Stewart in the Hill Country each year for several years. She would take us to dinner at the country club or the St. Anthony's Club. Ironically, her favorite drink was a champagne cocktail.

We would meet her at her house near the Trinity University campus. It was a beautiful Spanish-style house with Mexican tile floors covered with Persian rugs. She had a glass collection in a spindly Victorian display cabinet with a curved glass front that Letha always admired. When Marietta closed the house, she insisted that we drive to San Antonio to take the cabinet. When we arrived, she told us that she had just sold all the Persian rugs. We would have bought several if they had been available. Every Christmas, we always sent her a box of her favorite chocolate-dipped dried apricots from the Neiman Marcus catalog.

Shortly after they were married, my parents visited the family in San Antonio. Emma was still alive, and Effie and Herta were maids in the house. Instead of tea, they drank beer in the afternoon. My father was sent to the basement bar to draw a pitcher of beer. He was the only man in the house that afternoon, so it fell to him to pour the beer. Tanta Emma thought he was too careful pouring the beer. He poured it down the side of the glasses like most college students. She wanted hers with a head on it. She told him to "put a collar on it, German-style." She told him that she wanted to see the bubbles in the glass, not feel them in her stomach. He told me he felt like a country bumpkin in that sophisticated house. I think my mother had to coach him a lot.

My grandfather Bentzen taught him how to carve a beef roast and a turkey or chicken. My father always insisted on a long, very sharp knife when he carved. He would sharpen the knife with a steel just before starting to carve. The beef had to be sliced very thinly, but perfectly even in thickness and served to the plate with the carving knife and fork. He prided himself in making large thin slices of turkey breast. When he carved a turkey or chicken, he always used his special "game shears" to disjoint the bird.

I think that my father also learned to smoke cigars from my grandfather Bentzen. Granddad always smoked three cigars every day during the time I knew him. He always removed the band before smoking a cigar. He considered it low class to smoke a cigar with the band on it. He thought the only reason to keep the band on the cigar was to brag by showing off the brand. He was above that.

After Granddad retired, he would usually go by bus on weekdays to the Missouri Athletic Club for lunch at the founders' table and smoke a cigar after lunch. He would go up to the card room to play gin rummy with several men from the table until about four o'clock while they discussed the problems of the world. After the game broke up, he would smoke another cigar. He would return home by taking the Maryland streetcar. His maid would serve him dinner unless he was going out to a play or the symphony. After dinner, he would smoke his third cigar while he read or listened to records of classical music.

My grandmother Bentzen died before I was a year old, so I never knew her. They were driving from St. Louis to Normal to visit us when an oncoming car crossed the center of the road and hit them head-on. Grandmother died from the accident, and my grandfather was in the hospital for several weeks.

When Bruce and I were young, the family would go to St. Louis to visit the family. Granddad's maid, Mable, would take Bruce and me on a streetcar ride all over St. Louis while my mom and dad had a quiet afternoon talking with Granddad.

Several years after my grandmother died, Granddad gave up his house on Maryland Avenue and moved into an apartment in the Pierre Chateau apartments on Lindell Boulevard. It was always interesting to visit him there. There was a doorman and an elevator operator. At the Pierre Chateau, they were both Filipino. I learned that in St. Louis, in the fifties, Filipino employees were considered more prestigious than black employees. Dad was not impressed.

My uncle Roy, Mom's brother, and his wife Lucille (Aunt Lou) lived in Sappington, Missouri, a suburb of St. Louis. We always visited them when we came to see Granddad Bentzen. Aunt Lou had a son, Gary, by a previous marriage whom we considered a cousin. He was Bruce's age.

Uncle Roy and Aunt Lou led a flamboyant country club lifestyle, which my father did not approve. They ran with a wealthy set that Roy's income could not equal. Aunt Lou was always nagging my granddad to give them his money so they could keep up with the Busches. My grandfather knew August Busch, the owner of Budweiser, but did not like or associate with him.

Roy and Lou's friends would go to Mountain Shadows or Camelback Inn in Phoenix for February and/or March, so Roy and Lou would have to go there for one or two weeks. The rest of the year Lucille would play bridge all afternoon with her friends who all consumed three or more martinis during the afternoon. Their husbands would join them for drinks before going to the country club for more drinks and dinner.

My father rarely drank alcohol and then never more than one, so he considered them all to be alcoholics. Lucille always starved herself to remain thin. Bruce once described her legs as two snakes hanging out of a gunny sack. Dad got a laugh out of that.

Chapter 4

In Normal, my parents had a nice circle of friends, most of whom attended the Normal Presbyterian church. They were very close with the Longs (Lee and Sugar) who lived in the apartment across the hall from them, shortly after my parents were married. Sugar had given birth to two boys who were born with heart problems and died very young. They had one daughter, Mary Alice (whom everyone called Molly), who did not have heart problems. Molly was about the same age as my brother. She grew up to become homecoming queen of the University of Illinois.

My parents also did things with Les and Wilma Cornick who had a daughter, Connie, about a year older than Bruce, and another girl, Martha, a year older than me. Other members of the group included Aura and "Tuffy" King, Max and Bernice Orr, Ray and "Willy" Oaks, and Bill and Fran Scott.

One New Year's Eve, about 1938, Dr. Lynn TenEycke, a friend and local dentist who was also a musician, was leading the dance band for the Wildwood Country Club party. He dedicated the song "Stormy Weather" to my parents because they argued all the time. (Stormy Weather was written in 1933 by Herald Arlen and Ted Koehler and was first sung by Ethel Waters at the Cotton Club. It was a very popular tune in 1938.) Friends thought it fit my parents. Mom and Dad apparently argued a lot throughout their married lives. After that night, they called "Stormy Weather" their song.

Shortly after my brother, Bruce, was born in November of 1936, they moved from the apartment on Fell Avenue into a bungalow on Normal Avenue in the north end of Normal, very close to the apartment where they had lived with the Longs.

When Bruce was about twenty months old, he climbed into my father's car that was parked in the driveway. He opened Dad's medical bag that was on the backseat of the car. He found the medication holder, the fold-open box that was lined on both sides with long glass bottles with screw caps, which were full of pills. He opened the bottle with the shiny red pills and began to suck on them. They were sugar-coated strychnine tablets, used to treat heart disease. Apparently, strychnine is very bitter. When the sugar coating dissolved, the pills became bitter, so he spit most of them out.

When he was discovered in the car with the strychnine tablets, Dad did not know if he had swallowed any, so they rushed him to the hospital to have his stomach pumped. He survived, but my father always kept his medical bag locked after that. Bruce had just eaten a large bowl of homemade peach ice cream, which my mother claims played a big role in his survival.

Within a year or so after that episode, they moved again, into a two-story brick house on Main Street. They had a young woman living with them who was studying to be an elementary schoolteacher at Illinois State Normal University. She lived in the house with free room and board in exchange for child care and light housework. Carrie Mae "Casey" Irwin became a very good friend of the family, and she and her eventual husband, Art Kuchan, had a significant role in the raising of Bruce and me.

When my mother went to the hospital to have me, she cooked several meals for my father to eat for the days she was in the hospital. One of the things she cooked was a pork roast. Before she left, she pointed it out to Casey and told her that if she could not think of anything else to feed my father, she could serve the roast. When my mother returned from the hospital, she learned that my father had eaten pork roast for five days in a row and was very tired of it. He had not complained, but Casey never lived that down.

I was born in July of 1939, and we lived for five more years in that house. Main Street in Normal carried two very important highways, the famous US 66 and also US 51, called Main Street USA because it went up the middle of the country from the Gulf of Mexico to Lake Superior. Both went up Main Street all the way through town. We could sit on the front porch and watch the world go by.

Because of the teacher's college, the town of Normal was incorporated dry. (In those days, teachers were not supposed to drink or smoke tobacco, at least not in public.) Main Street went from Normal into Bloomington about one block from our house. Bloomington was wet. There were big signs hanging out as far as the law allowed over Main Street, advertising the liquor store on the west side of the street and the bar on the east side. Main Street started uphill in front of our house, so those signs were visible in Normal for several blocks.

Dad was in the military for three years while we lived in that house on Main Street. I remember large blocks of coal burning in the living room fireplace to heat the downstairs because the furnace was turned off. Coal was rationed because of the war, and it was expensive when it could be bought. Most local doctor's bills were paid to some extent with ration coupons during the war, but Dad was in the army and not practicing in Normal so we did not have extra coupons. Mom was upset about that because the other doctor's wives were able to buy all they wanted with the extra coupons.

One year, during my father's military absence, Lee Long played Santa Claus when he was home on leave. Other years, Mr. Von Fossen, who lived across Apple Street and had a natural white beard and a more Santa Claus physique, filled that role.

The first Steak 'n Shake was started in Normal, a block from our house. Gus Belt started the fast-food restaurant with the slogan "In sight, it must be right." There was a lunch counter inside from which you could see into the kitchen. No cook would dare to pick up a hamburger he had flipped onto the floor and put it back on the grill.

My father was Gus Belt's doctor and knew him well. My father told me that Gus had a gambling problem with the horses. He would go to Chicago to the racetrack and run up a gambling debt using the restaurant as collateral. Then he would have to give up the restaurant to settle his debts. The third time he started the restaurant, they put everything in his wife's name so he could not use it as collateral. Steak 'n Shake went on to be the multistate chain it is today.

It was a big outing when Dad took us to Steak 'n Shake. There was a big parking lot, and the food was served in the parking lot by curbies. The curbies would run from the kitchen with your food on a tray and hook it onto the window of your car. When you finished, you would honk the horn or flash your headlights, and a curbie would come to collect your payment and retrieve the tray. There were tables inside, but the point of going to Steak 'n Shake was to see and be seen in the parking lot.

When I was in high school, everyone would cruise Steak 'n Shake. When you learned to drive, one of the first things you wanted to learn was how to back into a parking place so you could watch everyone else who drove through. On busy nights, cars would circle through and go round and round. Since Steak 'n Shake was on Main Street with US 51 and 66 both going past, circling the parking lot involved going onto the highway and reentering the drive-in. Traffic would get jammed, so Bill Craig, the local cop, would have to come to direct traffic. If he saw you coming around for a second time, he sent you up Virginia Avenue, away from the traffic, and told you not to come back for at least fifteen minutes.

CHAPTER 5

MY FATHER WAS VERY PROUD of his membership as a fellow of the American College of Surgeons. Application to be invited to join the ACS involved having done many surgical operations and the review of a number of surgical cases of the applicant by the college examiners to determine whether standards were met.

When he applied for membership, another of the requirements was the publication of a scientific paper on a surgical subject in one of the major journals. He had published one paper. It was on the subject of removing tar from skin that had been burned by hot tar. Tar burns were a common injury in roofers and road workers. Removal of the burned tissue to allow healing and treatment of burns was the job of surgeons. Tar was difficult to separate from the skin and would retard the healing of burned skin if it were not removed. He discovered that rubbing Vaseline on the tar would dissolve the tar so it could be wiped from the skin. His paper on this was accepted for publication.

He applied to become a fellow of the American College of Surgeons in 1942 during his first year of military service while he was stationed at Camp Grant in Rockford, Illinois. The ACS is a very deliberative organization. He did not learn of his acceptance until the last days of his military service in 1945. By that time, he had added 1,308 surgical procedures, 3,850 X-ray readings, and 262 radiologic procedures including fluoroscopic exams, gastrointestinal series, and chest films to his pre military numbers. These were done at the 188th

Station Hospital at Narsarsuaq Army Air Base (Bluie East One, BE 1) where he also supervised the physiotherapy department and directed over 7,100 rehabilitation treatments in the clinic and on the wards.

His application to become a fellow in the American College of Surgery was accepted during his last month of military service. He was inducted into the college at the annual meeting in Chicago the next year. His pride in this recognition caused him to always add the "FACS" after his name when he signed anything medical. He eventually became program chairman and then president of the Illinois chapter of the American College of Surgeons in the mid-1950s. He was a one-on-one type of person, so for him to run an organization like this, he had to rely on his military experience and managed to pull it off. His year of being chief of surgery of the military hospital in Greenland was good preparation for his leadership role.

He was also elected president of the McLean County Medical Society. While he was president of the medical society, there was a new doctor in town who was called to see a very wealthy widow who lived in a castle, which was complete with a moat and drawbridge, located out past the edge of Bloomington.

She was having chest pain, which he diagnosed as angina. The new doctor gave her some nitroglycerin tablets that made the pain go away. He stayed for about half an hour to reassure her that she was not having a heart attack. Shortly thereafter that visit, the new doctor sent her a bill for $500. (My father was charging either $5 or $8 for house calls at that time.) She complained to the medical society.

My father told me that the executive board of the society called the doctor before them and asked him about the bill. He told them that he believed that he could and should charge rich people as much as they could pay. The society board did not agree: they told him to change his ways or move on down the road. He moved away and was immediately sued for breach of promise by three different women in Bloomington. The community was well rid of him.

In those days, the medical community disciplined itself. Now the legal profession has made that very difficult and bad doctors go undisciplined. The doctors who agree to serve on hospital and organization committees do not want to be sued for millions of dollars for carrying out the decisions of ethics committees. The Federal Trade Commission adds to the problem by filing suits against doctors on ethics committees, claiming restraint of commerce when a doctor is disciplined.

During Dad's presidency, he criticized a local osteopath. He described the treatment being given to a patient by the osteopath as being "asinine." The osteopath sued him and the County Medical Society for defamation and restraint of trade. I think this was finally settled out of court, but Dad never used the term "asinine" again. My father did not think that osteopaths were well trained in medicine and did not feel that physical manipulation was adequate therapy for most illnesses.

(Since then, the training of osteopathic physicians has improved dramatically. They still use physical manipulation to treat some diseases, but have incorporated allopathic [MD] medicine into their training. In Pittsburgh, I trained osteopathic physicians to be ophthalmologists and found them to be good physicians.)

(Every year, all residents in the United States who are in ophthalmology training take an "in service" examination that has no official licensing status and cannot be used in a punitive manner by the program director. This exam is graded on a percentile basis in comparison with every other ophthalmology resident in the country. It lets the individual know how they compare with all the other residents at their stage in training and prepares them for the Ophthalmology Board Examination that they will take at the end of their residency training. There is a section of this examination that tests knowledge of general medicine. On some years, the osteopathic physicians [DOs] in my program scored higher in that section that the allopathic physicians [MDs]. There were several American Ophthalmology Board Certified DO ophthalmologists on the teaching faculty at St. Francis Medical Center.)

(At the University of Texas Medical Branch in Galveston, I was not allowed to interview osteopathic physicians for residency positions, much less accept them for a position. I believe that this is a widely held position by allopathic medical school based residency programs.)

Chapter 6

By 1941, when the United States decided to get into World War II, my father had a busy practice and was doing surgery several days a week. We lived in the big brick house on Main Street. I was two years old, and Bruce had just turned five. My father drove a four-door Buick sedan, and my mother had a little blue Chevrolet coupe with a split bench seat in front and a platform in the back.

The milkman delivered milk to the back steps every day, and the coal man came about once a month during the winter to dump coal down a chute into the basement coal room. During the winter, the milk on the back steps froze and expanded, causing it to extrude from the neck of the bottle, lifting the waxed paper cap an inch or two above the rim of the bottle. Mom had to cut the frozen milk, or cream, off the bottle while it was frozen to melt in a bowl so it would not run down the outside of the bottle when it melted.

There was a horse-drawn ice wagon that came down the street every day. We had an electric refrigerator so we did not need ice, but many in the neighborhood still used iceboxes. The horse knew the route and would pull the wagon down the street and stop at the houses that bought ice, even when the driver was carrying ice to the last house and not in the driver's seat.

My father continued his lifelong joy of hunting. He knew many farmers who would allow him to hunt pheasants in the cornfields on their land. A group of doctors took an annual trip to southern

Arkansas rice country, near Stuttgart, to hunt ducks. They would wade in hip boots and pull johnboats into the flooded pin oak forests to hunt ducks over decoys in the flooded clearings within the forests.

The ducks would feed on the scattered rice in the harvested rice fields and fly to the ponds in the flooded sections of pin oak forests to rest. Dad had photographs of the six hunters with sixty ducks piled on a johnboat. The limit was ten ducks per hunter for the six hunters. He told me that they always had their limits by nine to ten o'clock in the morning. Then they would drink coffee and play cards for the rest of the day.

Dad was duck hunting along the Sangamon River in Western Illinois on December 7, 1941. When he came out of the duck blind and got back to civilization, everyone was honking their horns. He turned on his car radio and learned that the Japanese had attacked Pearl Harbor.

The army needed doctors after Pearl Harbor when the United States entered the war so they started a doctor draft. A doctor could be drafted until they were forty years old. My father was thirty-seven and worried that he could be drafted as a general doctor. Specialists were kept back at the army hospitals, but GPs like him were sent onto the battle fields, at or near the front, to accompany the medics.

Talking with other physicians at the hospital, he learned that a doctor could voluntarily enlist for nonoverseas duty, avoiding the risks of the battlefield. These positions were limited, so he decided that with a wife and two small children at home, he should enlist a soon as possible to get one of the nonoverseas positions. He went directly to the recruitment office to enlist and then went home to tell my mother about his good fortune of staying "nonoverseas."

My mother was not happy with his decision. I do not think she ever forgave him for enlisting. She told me just before she died that she thought it was the worst decision he ever made. I think Dad's war years were the zenith of his career.

Immediately after he enlisted, the community was declared to have a critical number of doctors, so no more doctors could be drafted. All the other doctors stayed home and practiced medicine. My mother was furious. He thought he was doing his patriotic duty.

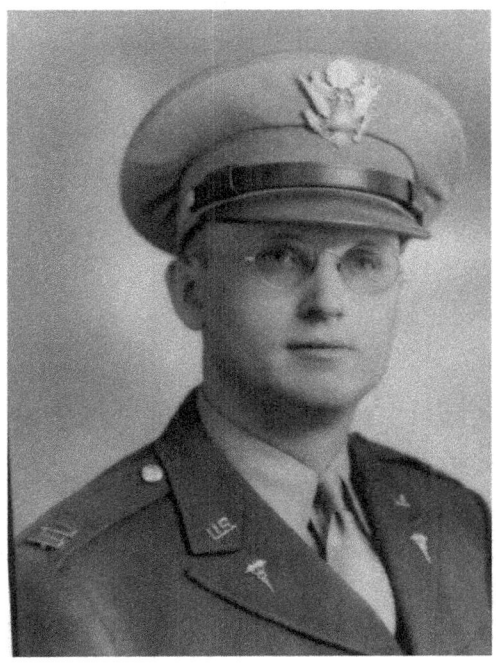

Captain Harry C. Barber in uniform, 1942.

My father was a captain in the army, stationed at first at Camp Grant in Rockford, Illinois, about one hundred and thirty-five miles from home. He was getting captain's pay and doing induction physical exams all day every day. Mom was left at home with two children to feed and look after.

The other doctors in Normal and Bloomington were busy practicing medicine in their offices and making a good income.

Patients often paid part of their bills with ration coupons for meat, sugar, coal, and gasoline, so the doctors were eating and living well. My father's patients were all young GIs who did not have ration coupons and did not pay the doctor anyway.

Dad had his car at Camp Grant so he sometimes came home on weekends. He would give rides to other officers who lived along the way. The older soldiers with families would pay him for the ride in ration coupons, usually gasoline coupons, so he kept his car in gas and gave some to my mother.

My father enjoyed his time at Camp Grant. He had regular hours; well patients, except for trauma from training; and was well fed. The doctors had an officer's club and sports facilities to enjoy during their off hours. He liked to play baseball with the officers when they were not working.

He especially liked the travel. Every troop train was required to have a doctor or two, depending on the number of soldiers on board. After basic training, the soldiers from Camp Grant went by train to New Orleans or the West Coast to ship out. He loved to ride the trains. Being the train doctor, he had free roam of the train and often passed the time talking with the conductors, riding on the back platform of the train. He told me that he went through every railroad mountain pass in the Rocky Mountains because the trains varied their routes to prevent espionage. He would chat with the conductors who knew the routes and told him where he was. He often traded these trips with other doctors who did not want to travel.

On one trip to New Orleans, he was supervising a troop train with another doctor who was from Kentucky and had an appreciation for good bourbon. Many of the troop trains had club cars that were available to the officers. Mississippi was a dry state, so they had to close the club car and lock up the whiskey while they were in Mississippi.

The Kentucky doctor had an attack of chest pain, just after they entered Mississippi, so the conductor called my dad to see him. Since all the soldiers were young and healthy, the doctors did not carry medicines for angina and heart attacks. The train did not have any of these medications either. My father told the conductor that the only thing available that would help his fellow doctor was some kind of drinkable alcohol to make his coronary arteries dilate.

The conductor left them and returned in a few minutes with two miniatures of bourbon from the club car—for medicinal use. The ailing doctor drank both bottles and said that it relieved his pain. The conductor then slipped my father two more miniature bottles of bourbon "in case the pain returned" or for his own consumption. I think my father drank the bourbon or split it with the Kentucky doctor. I was never sure when my father told that story that the Kentucky doctor's chest pain was real.

Chapter 7

After more than a year at Camp Grant, Dad received orders to prepare for a cold, damp climate, but no specific location. He went to the quartermaster to get cold-weather uniforms. He had several days to report to Taunton, Massachusetts, to ship out to his "nonoverseas" assignment. Because of the secrecy of the war, they would not tell him where he was going until they were offshore. My mother went with him to Taunton and left Bruce and me with "Auntie Parker," an elderly woman who often babysat the two of us.

My father loved to fish and thought that a cold, damp climate might have some good places to fish. He went to the post exchange (PX) and bought two fishing rods, a fly rod and a casting rod. These rods could be taken apart for travel and were in aluminum traveling tubes, but it was obvious what they were. He carried them up the gangplank while most of his fellow physicians were carrying all the whiskey they could manage, supposedly to ward off the cold weather.

He spent almost thirty days on a troop ship in the North Atlantic Ocean to get to his "nonoverseas" duty post. They were in convoy of over fifty ships with blimps overhead much of the time to spot enemy submarines. Because he was a physician and an officer, he had better housing on the ship. The physicians and other officers shared staterooms. The GIs had tiered bunks in large rooms.

The handles were removed from all the shower faucets because of limited water supply for the number of soldiers on the ship. This did not bother my father and his roommates because my father always carried a pair of pliers with him when he traveled. They used his pliers to turn on and off the faucets to shower every few days.

The other problem with the staterooms was that the ship had debarkation nets hung on the sides in case they were hit by a torpedo and had to quickly abandon ship. He told me that the porthole for their stateroom would open and was large enough for them to crawl through, but the netting was in front of the porthole. As an officer, he was allowed to carry a weapon, so he put on his belt knife with a sharp six-inch blade to have it handy if they needed to cut the netting to escape through the porthole. Fortunately, they did not have to abandon ship.

Dad always carried a sharp penknife with two blades in his pocket. He made sure that it was always very sharp, so I am sure that his belt knife on that ship had a very sharp blade.

His group of physicians and hospital personnel was dropped off on the east coast of Greenland before the convoy proceeded to Europe with the main body of troops. He found himself at an army air corps airport with a 250-bed hospital and barracks for the doctors, nurses, and other hospital personnel. The camp had other support buildings. This base was near Narsarsuaq, the Eskimo settlement on the southeast coast of Greenland near the Arctic Circle. He was one of several doctors whose duty was to patch, repair, and rehabilitate sick or wounded soldiers from the European war theater.

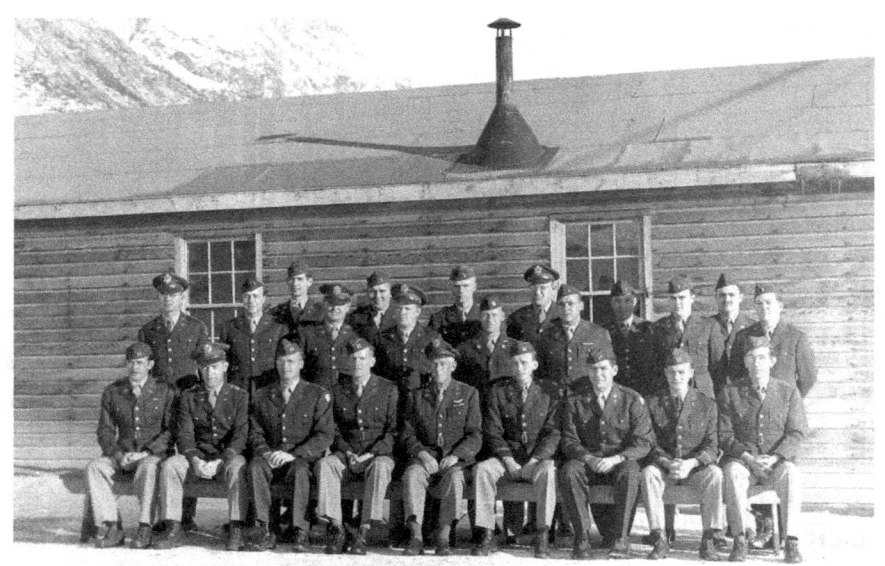

Medical Officers assigned to Army
base BE2 (Bluie East 2) in 1943

The soldiers were flown in, operated, and rehabilitated at the hospital until they were ready to be sent back to Europe to rejoin their units or fill in other units. Under the existing army regulations, if your injury was treatable within the battle theater, you could be sent back to your unit. The east coast of Greenland was considered within the battle theater. (German submarines, U-boats, roamed the North Atlantic and mined the coast of Greenland.) If the injury was significant and required extensive rehab or rendered the soldier unable to return to combat, they were flown back to the United States to receive treatment, their Purple Heart, and a medical discharge.

In the war, there were periods of relative calm punctuated by intense battles with enough injuries to fill the four military hospitals on the east coast of Greenland. At times, they were very busy with all operating rooms in use. In between battles, the doctors made rounds and helped the patients rehabilitate. When the patients had been shipped out, the doctors had lots of time on their hands. They learned board games, took up wood and metalworking hobbies, and sought recreation, either in the Quonset hut or outdoors.

There were several doctors and other personnel who were Master Masons, so Dad organized the Arctic Circle Masonic Club and served as president of the club.

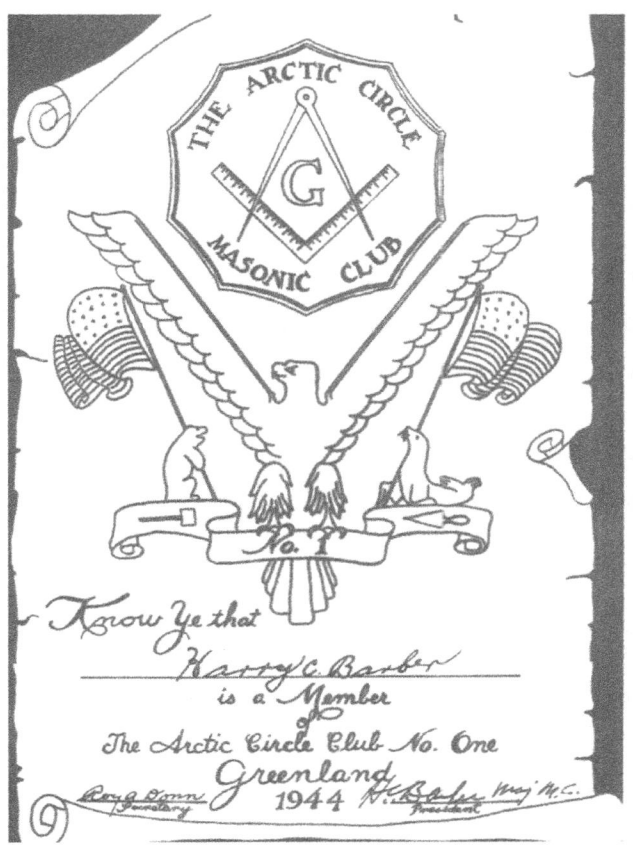

Harry Barber's Arctic Circle Masonic Club No. One Certificate, 1944.

My father learned to play cribbage and became the hospital cribbage champion. Dad loved fresh tomatoes, so he wrote home asking for tomato seeds to grow tomatoes in one corner of the recreation Quonset hut, using 60-watt light bulbs for sunshine during the long Arctic midnight. He told me that he grew several plants, but they would not set tomatoes. He soon realized that there were no insects during the winter in this icy climate to pollinate the blossoms, so he used cotton-tipped applicators from the hospital to hand pollinate the blossoms. He soon had a good crop of green tomatoes.

After one crop, he gave up on growing tomatoes. He told me that as soon as the green tomato began to show an orange or pink blush, the tomato would disappear. The other doctors blamed it on the raccoons, but my father said he never saw a four-legged raccoon while he was in Greenland, especially not inside the Quonset hut. He never learned who was taking the tomatoes.

We have a family heirloom that my father made while he was in Greenland. It is a huge carving knife. The blade was made from a band saw blade, and the handle was made of successive rings of aluminum and various colors of the plastic that was recovered from damaged gun turrets of American bombers. The blade is about two inches wide and twelve inches long with rows of circular whorl marks on both sides, made by pressing a dowel rod in a drill press against the steel blade coated with wet pumice. There is a four-inch-wide aluminum bar between the blade and handle. The knife is big, but light, and it does a good job carving long thin slices from a Thanksgiving turkey. The aluminum and plastic handle makes it surprisingly light and well balanced.

When the ice melted in the spring (June), there were salmon and halibut to be caught in the fjord next to the hospital and in the streams that flowed into it. My father got the chance to use his fishing rods. The other doctors who had taken whiskey to the cold, damp climate and laughed at his fishing rods now wanted to borrow the fishing rods.

There were no fishing rods or lures at the small base PX, so they had to improvise. They stole spoons from the cafeteria and took them to the machine shop to cut off the handles. They drilled two holes in the bowl of the spoon, one at each end. My father wrote home asking for fishing leaders and treble fishing hooks to be included in his next "care package" from home. He hooked the leader to the hole in the small end of the spoon and wired the hooks to the other end of the spoon bowl. He used his fly rod to catch salmon going up the streams. To fish through the ice for halibut, they used the modified kitchen spoons or used strings of tin foil taken from chewing gum wrappers, hung on the hooks, and tied the hooks on the line.

In the fall and early winter, Dad liked to hunt ptarmigan and eider ducks along the fjords. In the summer, he tried his hand at the Eskimo kayak and swimming in the ice-cold water of the fjord. During the winter, they had dogsleds and used the Eskimo dogs. They had both Alaskan and Greenland sleds. The Alaskan sleds ran a double string of dogs, but the Greenland Eskimos used a fan harness with the dogs all running side by side.

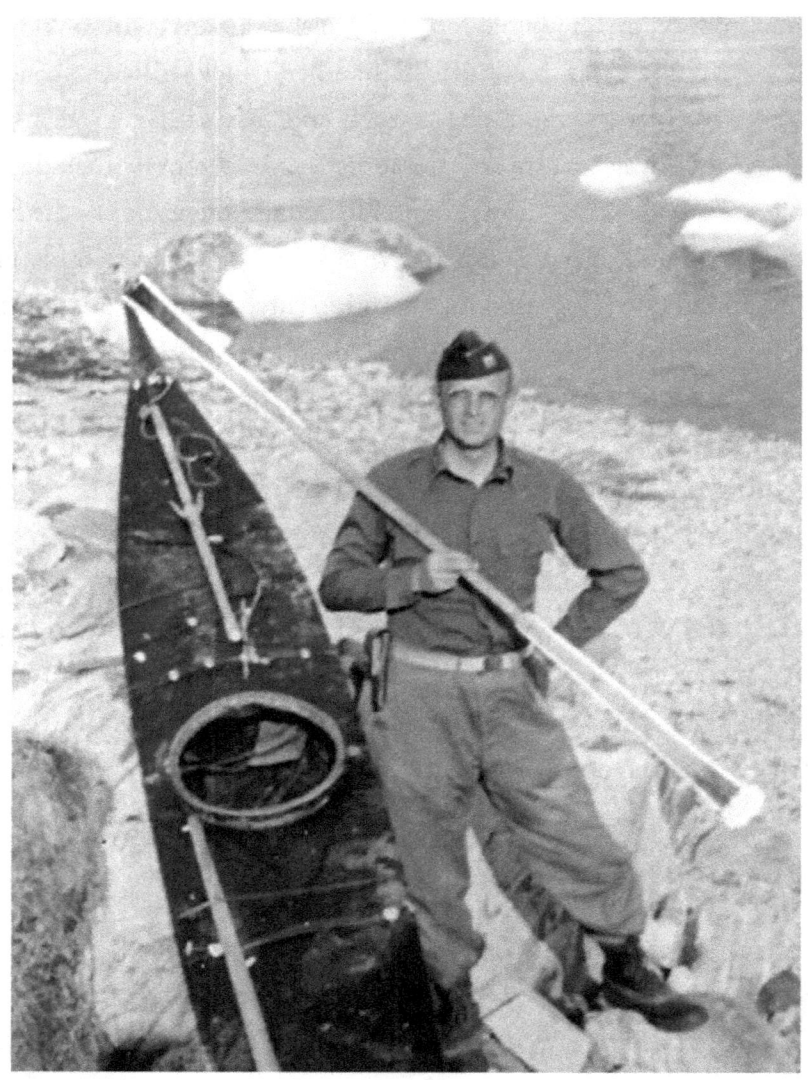

Harry Barber with Eskimo Kayak at BE2.

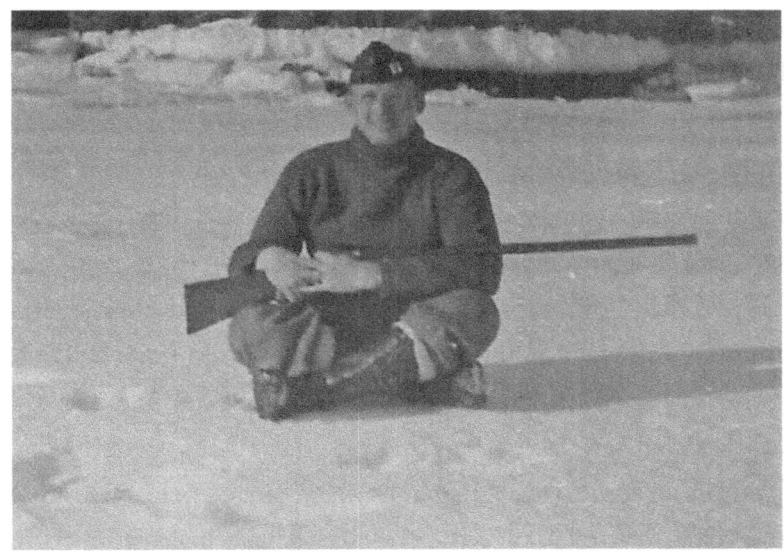

Harry Barber sitting on the ice with a shotgun ready to hunt Ptarmigan.

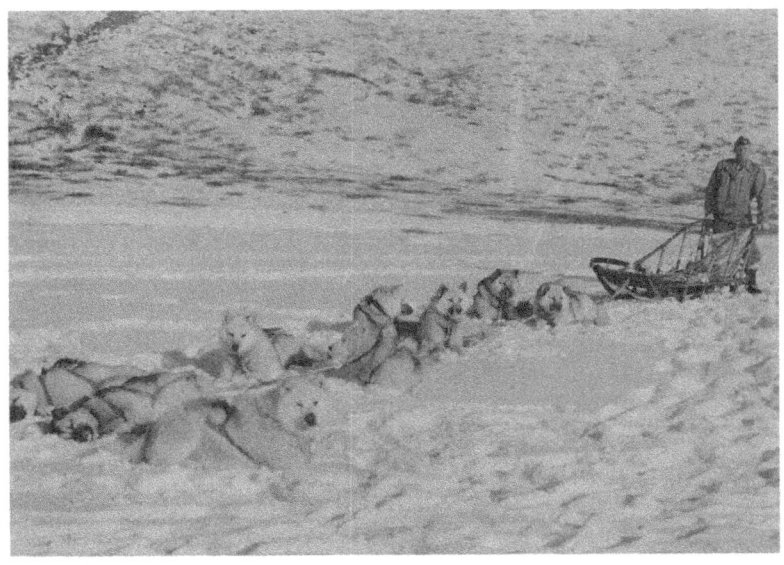

Harry Barber with Eskimo dog sled with American harness.

There was a hill behind the hospital, so the army sent in some wooden skis—standard government issue, meant for cross-country skiing. The soldiers wore their combat boots and strapped the skis to their boots with leather straps that went through slots in the skis—definitely not quick-release bindings. Always adventuresome, my father tore a knee cartilage when he fell while trying to ski down that hill. He had to use a cane for a while, but it did not keep him from doing surgery.

There is a photograph of a group of doctors and nurses gathered around a piano with one of the doctors playing the piano. Dad said that they often did this after dinner. Although no one had a great voice, they had fun trying. Another photo shows some of the doctors and nurses decorating a Christmas tree. Since there were no trees in that part of Greenland, the tree must have been shipped in for the hospital. The doctors and nurses developed a sense of family to counteract the isolation of Greenland.

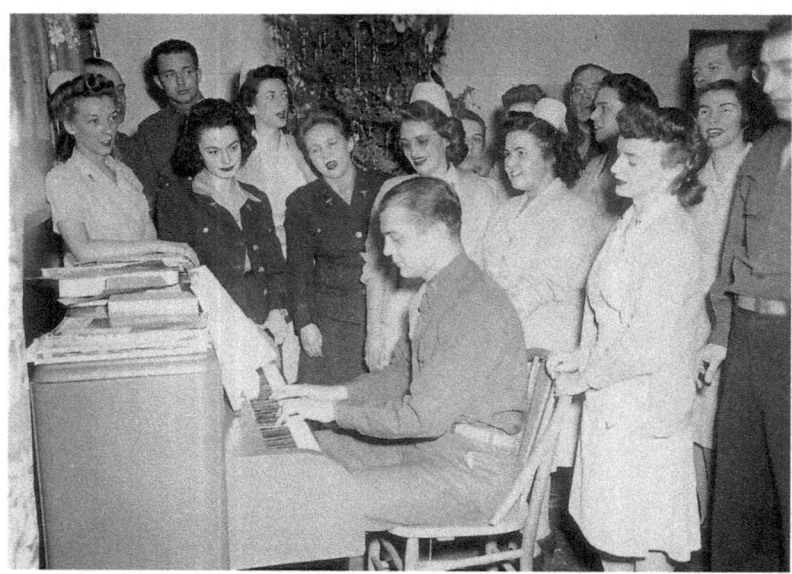

Base personnel gathered around the
piano singing Christmas Carols.

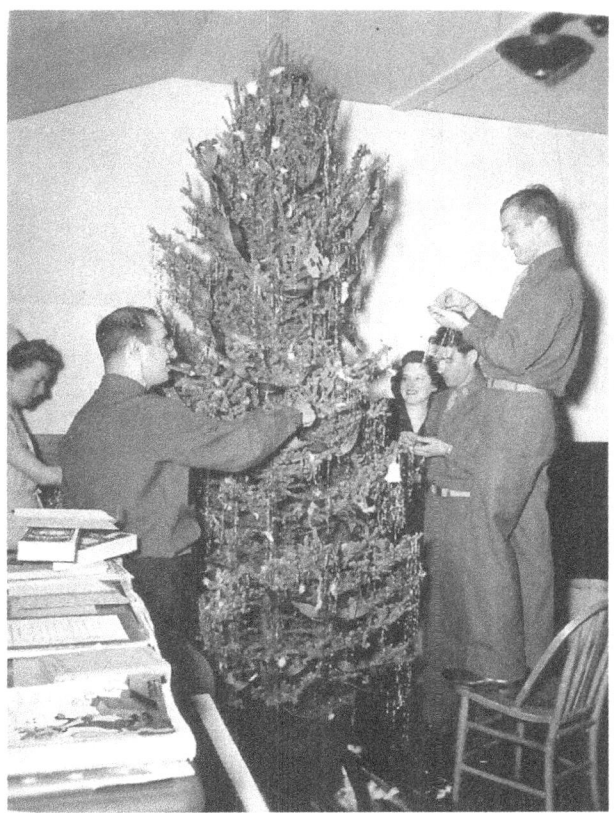

Doctors and nurses decorating the
hospital Christmas tree.

My mother shipped a record player and a box of phonograph records to Dad. He often remarked in his letters home that the staff spent evenings listening to the records when the northern lights interfered with shortwave reception so badly that they could not understand what was being said. New shipments of records were always appreciated.

Occasionally, a patrol boat would stop at the base for a visit. If things were slow, they would take the officers on rides up the fjords to see the Eskimo villages and watch parts of the glaciers break off into the fjord to make icebergs. He found the natives to be very friendly people who doted on their children and loved to show off their skills with kayaks and hunting weapons.

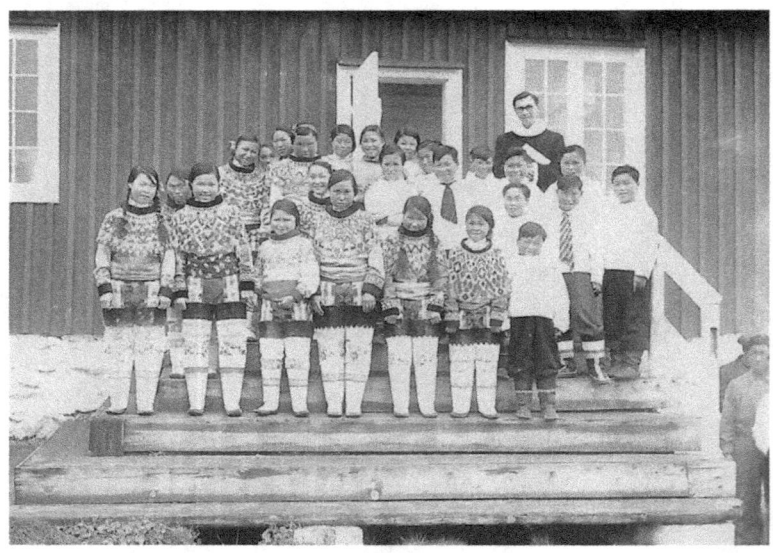

Eskimo children in native dress with missionary on the steps of the Danish church school.

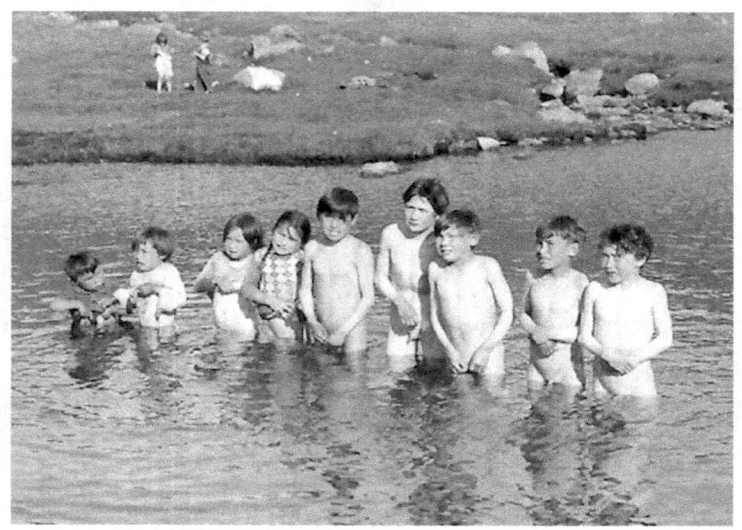

Eskimo children standing in icy cold water in Sondrestrom Fjord, Greenland.

The standard tour of duty at these remote hospitals in Greenland was eight months. At the end of eight months, my father prepared to be relieved of duty and reassigned stateside. Under standard operating procedures, an officer could not leave his duty post until he was relieved of duty by his successor. His successor never arrived. The replacement had apparently pulled some strings and gotten reassigned elsewhere. "The brass" informed my father that he was extended in Greenland for eight more months.

Shortly after that, he was promoted from captain to major and sent to another Greenland military hospital to be the chief of surgery. This hospital was near Ammassalik on Scoresby Sound, the largest fjord system in the world. When he arrived, he learned that the hospital was a mess and that the previous chief of surgery had been relieved of duty for incompetence. Dad continued to do surgery and practice medicine while running the medical staff. He had administrative officers to handle the nuts and bolts while he ran the staffing.

He enjoyed a few perks as chief of surgery. One of the things he enjoyed the most was getting to know Captain Bob Bartlett, the captain of the Newfoundland schooner, *Ellie M. Morrissey*. My father liked to tell everyone about his visits with Bartlett.

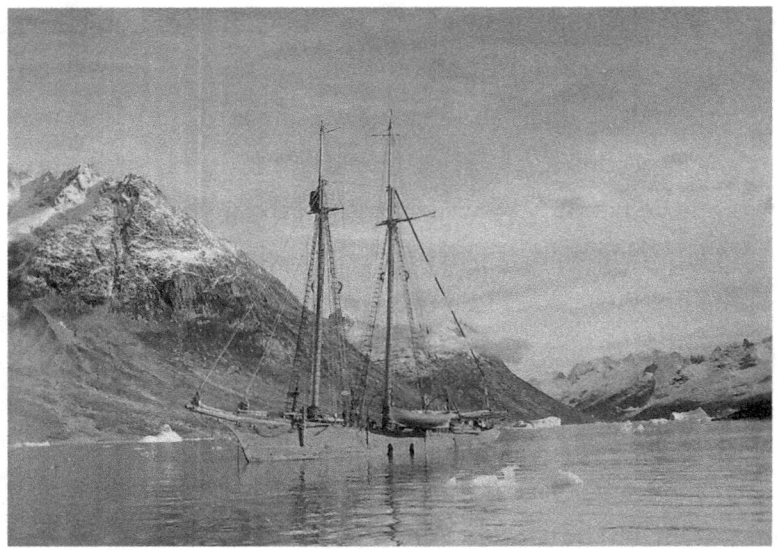

The Newfoundland schooner *Ellie M. Morrissey*, Bartlett's ship, at anchor at BE2.

The wooden schooner was used as a supply ship to the hospitals along the coast. Dad told me that the Germans had mined the coast of Greenland with magnetic ocean mines to interrupt the work of the hospitals and air bases. The United States often used wooden ships to supply the bases because they would not set off the magnetic mines.

When Bartlett arrived at the hospital, he would send a message ashore to invite the officers to his boat for tea. My father would often go out to the ship to join Bartlett. Bartlett and my father were both storytellers. They would sit for hours and swap stories, often through dinner aboard ship, if my father did not have pressing duties.

Bartlett kept a library of books on his schooner, most of them about Arctic exploration. He invited my father to come aboard to read the books whenever he was in port. Bartlett never knew when he might get orders to heave anchor and leave immediately, so he did not allow his books to leave the ship.

Bartlett had been the sea captain of the schooner *Roosevelt* that took Robert Perry to the north on his discovery of the North Pole in 1909. My father told me that Bartlett was a staunch defender of Perry when Frederick Cook made his claim of having beaten Perry to the pole. Perry had taken Cook north on prior expeditions and dropped him off in Greenland again, on his way to discover the North Pole. Bartlett believed that Cook wintered in a cave on Ellesmere Island with two Eskimos before returning to Greenland with them and that he had made up the story of his trip to the North Pole. One reason for this disbelief was that Cook had described a mountain range near the pole that has never been seen by other explorers before or since that time, even with modern satellites. Some people believe that Cook killed one of the two Eskimos and that the other was later proven to be a serial liar.

Cook's claim to be the first and fastest to scale Mount McKinley in Alaska has also been disproven. The photographic negative that had been used to make the print to prove that Cook was at the top of McKinley was discovered. The print from the negative had been cropped to show Cook on top of Mount McKinley. The original uncropped negative showed a taller mountain behind him.

Bartlett was somewhat disenchanted by Perry and had some doubts whether Perry had actually reached the pole. Bartlett told my father that he (Bartlett) led the expedition north from his ship, hacking the trail through ice ridges with the advance party. Perry would follow behind on the improved trail and arrive after the next camp was set up, usually retiring into an igloo that had been prepared for him. He insisted that he had to be well rested and have the freshest dogs for the final dash to the pole so others had to do the hard work of getting him there.

When they were near the pole, Perry sent Bartlett back to the ship with everyone in the party except four Eskimos and his black valet. The expedition was organized in groups of three, one leader with two Eskimos.

Perry's reasoning, stated in his own book, was that Bartlett was second in command and would need to get everyone else back home if Perry vanished on his final dash to the pole and the subsequent return to the ship. Bartlett confided in my father that he thought Perry wanted to be the first and only white man to the pole.

Bartlett told Dad that Perry had torn two pages from his bound logbook on which he recorded his instrument sightings that proved he had reached the pole. Perry later copied the data into the logbook from the two pages after he had checked the sightings and calculations when he was back aboard the ship. Bartlett was not sure whether he copied the original readings from the loose pages or some mathematically corrected numbers.

Perry's average travel with the expedition, before his last sprint to the pole, was fifteen miles a day. For Perry to have reached the pole when he said he did, he had to average thirty miles a day after Bartlett and the rest of the expedition turned back to the ship. Perry had only six men and two sleds on the last dash, so it is possible that he did make such good time across smooth ice.

From reading Perry's account of his dash to the pole, I believe that he thought he was at the pole. He took sightings with a sextant using an artificial horizon for accuracy. He traveled in all four directions from the pole in case he was slightly off. Of course, once you believe that you have arrived, there is no point in going further, so he raced back to the ship before the ice broke up as summer approached.

Some believe that the distance from the pole to the ship was too far to have been traveled in the time Perry said he made the trip.

When Bartlett defended Perry against Cook's claim of beating Perry to the North Pole, he argued that it was possible under the excellent weather and ice conditions that happened to exist at the time.

The North Pole is within the Arctic Ocean, covered with ice that shifts constantly. Nansen proved that the ice cap rotates and part of it moves south toward Greenland. Debris from shipwrecks north of Siberia has been found in the North Atlantic. When Nansen tried to dash across the ice to the pole from his farthest north in the *Fram*, he learned that the ice drifted south faster than he could dogsled north. This rotation could have speeded Perry's return from the pole.

Bartlett was an old salt from Brigus, Newfoundland. He told my father about some of his trips for fishing and seal hunting and his voyages of Arctic exploration. He searched for specimen animals and sea creatures for museums and zoos and took Boy Scout groups and sons of his wealthy financial backers along for the adventure. One of his most memorable trips was a scientific expedition to explore the Arctic Ocean north of Alaska. Bartlett's book, *The Last Voyage of the Karluk*, describes the survival of the men on board the *Karluk* when the ship was crushed by ice and sank in 1913. This was one of the books my father read aboard the *Morrissey*.

My father tried to photograph the northern lights, but the mail was all censored by the army. In those days, he had to send the film to Kodak in the United States for processing. When the mounted slides were sent back to him, none of the photographs of the northern lights made it past the censors. Pictures of the hospital, the other doctors and nurses, and the glaciers near the base, all made it through. The northern lights are so random and the patterns so evanescent that they would not give any clue where the photographs were taken. My father thought that some censor now has some good pictures of the northern lights. I can also remember seeing holes in his letters home where whole sentences had been cut out with a razor blade. My mother kept his letters all of her life, and I have them now.

I have seen old 16mm movies that Dad made of the doctors fishing, rowing boats, paddling kayaks, and skinny dipping near floating ice on the Fourth of July. He also took movies of the natives rolling their kayaks over in the icy water. He took wonderful movies of the huge glaciers, showing large chunks of ice breaking off and falling into the water below. I believe that he sent the movies to Kodak for processing and Kodak sent them on to my mother, so they did not get censored.

One of my father's favorite stories was about the military hospitals providing medical care to the Eskimos. A boy, about ten years old, was brought to the hospital with a stiff neck and headache while my father was covering the emergency service. These were early signs of meningitis, so my father decided they needed to do a lumbar puncture (spinal tap) to confirm the diagnosis.

The usual way to do a lumbar puncture on a child is for a seated doctor or nurse to hold the child wrapped around the holder's abdomen with the child's head and shoulders under one arm and their legs under the other arm. Another doctor then places the needle into the spinal column between two vertebrae in the lower spine. Normal spinal fluid is clear. If it is milky, the child has meningitis.

My father and the other doctor flipped a coin to see who would hold the child and who would insert the needle. My father won the toss and elected to put the needle in. When he stuck the needle in the child's spine, the child bit the other doctor on his side, just below the ribs. It was all the doctor could do to continue to hold the child in position. The spinal fluid that came out of the needle was milky white, so they knew immediately that he had meningitis.

They had just received a shipment of a new antibiotic called penicillin G, which was being used by the army doctors to fight any and all infections. Without removing the needle from the spine, my father drew up a vial of penicillin into a syringe and shot it in through the needle that was already in his spine. (I have been told that this is not a presently approved method of treating meningitis.)

Iggy, that was the boy's hospital name, recovered over the next two weeks, but by that time, the Arctic winter had set in and they could not return the child to his village. They gave the child his own room to sleep in and made him an orderly. He rapidly learned enough English to be helpful and became a pet project of the nurses.

By the time they could return him to his village, it was six months later and he was fairly fluent in English. My father made a list of medical terms and sat down with Iggy to match the English terms with Eskimo words that my father wrote down phonetically. They posted this list in all the examination rooms, where it was a tremendous help to the doctors trying to treat the natives.

The military hospitals were always plagued by lack of supplies. At one time, they had a shortage of Novocain to use for local anesthesia. They used it to numb around a laceration or do a local nerve block before placing stitches to close a wound. Dad developed a technique to use saline to put pressure on nerves to block nerve conduction to numb an area for repair. He knew where nerves went under ligaments in the fingers and hands and was able to inject the saline under the ligament to create enough pressure to block the nerve conduction long enough to suture a cut or remove a wart. This allowed him to save the Novocain for other procedures.

The army doctors did not accept any pay for the care provided to the natives, but the people brought gifts of local crafts to them. By the time he was finally relieved of duty in Greenland, my father had a collection of common, dress, and wedding mukluks (Eskimo shoes), carved ivory from walrus and narwhale tusks, eiderdown baby blankets, and beautifully detailed kayak models made from bones and seal skin. He also brought home a baby polar bear skin that measured six feet across the back, from claw to claw on the forelegs. Soldiers were not allowed to hunt polar bears, but they could buy bear skins from the Eskimos. Dad bought one and shipped it home to have it tanned and finished as a rug with a mounted head.

Dad said that occasionally the soldiers who were standing guard at the base perimeter would see a group of Eskimo men tracking a bear. They would shoot the bear and leave it for the approaching hunters to clean for the meat and skin. The Eskimos would use many of the body parts for clothing, tools, bags, and igloo windows.

When his second eight months concluded, he packed up to come home, but his replacement did not arrive this time either. He was stuck for another eight months. This really bothered my mother, but I think my dad was in his element patching up wounded soldiers.

Much of what he did involved fixing fractures from bullet wounds and shrapnel. Repairing injuries often requires innovative procedures and reconstruction, which he loved. Many of the bones had to be stabilized with metal bone plates and screws. When he arrived in Greenland, the army had supplied the hospitals with nickel bone plates and brass screws. He remembered high school chemistry experiments using nickel and brass plates to make batteries and demonstrate electrolytic corrosion. He immediately requested that the army supply them with either nickel screws or brass plates so the screws would match the plates and would not corrode the screws to loosen the plates.

One of my father's favorite stories from Greenland was about a planeload of soldiers in a DC-4 that stopped in the Greenland base to refuel on the way to Europe. The DC-4 airplane was supported by two wheels under the wings and a nose wheel. While The DC-3 sat with the tailskid on the ground and had a foldout stairway, the DC-4 stayed horizontal with the door high above the ground. The soldiers needed a ladder or stairway to deplane.

The pilot had taxied the plane next to a large snowdrift near the terminal. One of the GIs decided not to wait for the ladder, but jumped into the snowdrift. The GI did not know that the snow had compacted into solid ice with an inch of new snow on the surface. He landed flat footed, expecting to sink into the snow. Instead, he fractured both heels on impact. Eight GIs jumped before they figured out what was happening and got the jumping stopped.

My father suddenly had eight cases of bilateral heel fractures to treat. He had not done this particular procedure of reducing heel fractures and stabilizing them with pins through the heel bone into the ankle although he had done all the elements of the procedure. He looked up the particulars in the orthopedic surgery books in the hospital library and went to work to pin and cast them all.

When the army received the report of eight bilateral heel fractures, they flew an orthopedic surgeon into Greenland to check the results. The orthopedist checked the patients and the post-pinning X-rays and congratulated my father that they were all done correctly. Then he told my father that he, as an orthopedist, had not done eight bilateral heel fracture repairs himself in his practice.

After many false starts and delays, the army assigned a replacement for him. A few weeks later, the war in Europe ended (May 7, 1945). The army put all replacements and reassignments on hold. Several weeks later, Dad was informed that he would be replaced in July. Near the end of his third eight-month stint, his orders finally came through to leave Greenland. His orders said that he did not have to wait for his replacement, who had already been delayed several times. Once Dad left, they would have to get his replacement to Greenland.

On his final day, he signed out and went down to the airstrip where he found a transport plane that was going back to the States empty, with the first stop in Boston. There were no seats in this cargo plane, so he found a pile of burlap sacks in the hangar and threw them into the cargo space with his duffle bag. He slept on the sacks during the flight to Boston.

CHAPTER 8

As he told the story, he caught a train from Boston to his next assignment. He was not given leave between assignments because he was needed at another hospital. However, I learned from his letters to Mom that he did not report to his next assignment until August. He describes his route to the new hospital in a letter to her as going through Decatur, Illinois, and Indianapolis, Indiana, to Charleston, West Virginia. From there, he "took 60 to the hospital gate." He would not have been in Decatur, Illinois, unless he had been in Normal. I was five years old then, but I do not remember his being home.

Someone must have felt guilty because of his triple stint in the Arctic. His next assignment was to do orthopedic and plastic surgery for repair and reconstruction of war injuries at the Ashford General Hospital. This was a hotel that had been converted to a military hospital. In peacetime, it was known as the Greenbrier Hotel at White Sulfur Springs, West Virginia, a luxury five-star, purchased by the government from the Chesapeake and Ohio Railroad. During the war, not many people were going to luxury hotels, so the railroad sold it to the army to use as a hospital. The rooftop solarium, with its big windows, had been converted into a series of operating rooms because of the available natural light.

When my father arrived, he learned that they were not expecting him until the next day. The officers, who were leaving for other assignments, had not left their rooms, so there was no vacant room for him in the bachelor officer's quarters. The only space available was the VIP suite above the front entrance of the hotel (the side entrance the last time I was there). They put him there as a temporary solution until a bachelor officer quarters room became available. Apparently, they forgot about him being in the VIP suite because he stayed there for several months until he was discharged from the army.

He told me that the doctors would operate every workday until they ran out of sterile instruments. They used a special type of dermatome to remove donor skin for skin grafts to cover burns and revise old burn scars. These dermatomes used a "drum" to hold the skin as it was removed. The sterilization of these drums took overnight, so when the doctors ran out of sterile drums, they had to quit.

Dad had free time in the evenings and on the weekends, which he spent using the Greenbrier facilities. There were two eighteen-hole golf courses, many tennis courts, big indoor and outdoor swimming pools, and a golf coffee shop that had been converted into an officer's club.

My father loved to swim, so he used the beautiful tiled indoor pool when he could. He believed that every man should know how to swim, especially soldiers. He was amazed at the number of soldiers who could not swim. He managed to obtain a key to the pool and began offering swimming classes. These were late in the afternoon, three days a week, and open to any soldiers wanting to learn to swim, if they were not in a cast or healing a fresh wound.

Shortly after Dad reported to his new assignment, Mom put my brother and me in her two-door blue Chevy coupe and headed for West Virginia. Her car had a split-backed front bench seat and a platform behind the seat. Sometimes we boys rode up front with

Mom, and sometimes we stretched out with a blanket and pillow on the platform. I remember staying in a tourist home in a residential neighborhood that I think was in Cincinnati, Ohio. This trip was the first time I had seen mountains, but they grew corn in the valleys of West Virginia, just like Illinois. There were no interstate highways, so the roads were crooked and steep.

We stayed two weeks in an apartment over the drugstore in White Sulfur Springs and visited the Greenbrier a lot. When my father learned that I did not know how to swim, he took me to the Greenbrier pool and taught me how to "dog-paddle" and float on my back.

There were large rooms on the main floor of the hotel that were filled with pool tables and ping-pong tables. These were busy with soldiers who were playing pool and ping-pong while dressed in hospital garb or fatigues and various casts. When I visited the Greenbrier years later, I learned that these were the lobby rooms of the hotel that were usually furnished with beautiful chairs, sofas, antique writing desks, and board game tables with inlaid woods to create the backgammon and chessboard patterns. As a hotel, the rooms were decorated with fine art on the walls and heavy curtains at the windows.

My father liked to play golf and had somehow acquired a set of clubs. On his afternoons off, my brother and I would carry his golf bag as he played the Old White Course. We noticed that there were many men grooming the golf courses, planting flowers, trimming hedges, and mowing grass. They all wore khaki pants and shirts with POW written on the front and back of their shirts. My dad explained that they were German prisoners of war. They lived in a tent city near the airport on the edge of the Greenbrier property and maintained the property of the Greenbrier.

Dad told me later that when the war was over, the POWs did not want to go back to war-torn Germany, but wanted to stay in the United States. Only when faced with repatriation did they try to escape from the fenced-in tent city.

I have seen a photograph of me, at the age of five, at the officer's club. My dad is holding me in his arms so that I could reach the arm of a slot machine. In my other hand, I am holding a glass of yellow liquid with a foamy white layer on the top. I do not recall getting to drink any of the liquid or pull the arm of the one-armed bandit, but I think the photo could get my parents in trouble today for corruption of a minor.

We went back home to go to school, and my father stayed at Ashford General Hospital for several months. Dad told me that while he was there, the American Board of Plastic Surgery held the plastic surgery board examinations at Valley Forge, Pennsylvania. All the surgeons at Ashford General had been doing the latest procedures in plastic surgery, so they wanted to sit for the board exam. My father volunteered to stay at the hospital to cover it while the others went to take the exam.

He explained to me that he knew that when he returned to Normal, Illinois, after the war, he would not need a shingle on the wall from the American Board of Plastic and Reconstructive Surgery to continue to do the procedures he had learned in the army. I think that by the number of times he told me that story, he actually missed having that shingle on his wall to remind him of his war years and the creative surgery that he had to do to repair war injuries. Dad was always very humble about things like this.

Years later when I visited the Greenbrier with my parents, my father told me that General Jonathan Wainwright, the hero of Bataan and Corregidor, had been brought there after the war while he was stationed there. Wainwright had lost so much weight from starvation and illness during the Bataan death march and the captivity afterward that he weighed less than one hundred pounds and was very weak. They put him in the Presidential Cottage with round-the-clock nurses and a Greenbrier chef to prepare anything and everything he wanted to eat, anytime he wanted it. He was in such bad physical shape from the march and the miserable prisoner-of-war camp conditions with accompanying diseases that he never fully recovered. He had been tortured and had suffered from repeated attacks of dysentery. Even with the heroic efforts to cure him after the war, he never regained his weight and health before he died in 1953.

In the 1980s, when I leased a Toyota Supra as a university perk, Dad was very upset with me. He told me that I should never buy anything from Japan because of what they did to "Skinny" Wainwright. He still thought that the Japanese were savages.

Chapter 9

After the war ended, my father spent several more months at Ashford General Hospital repairing poorly healed fractures, transplanting tendons to reroute muscle groups, and grafting skin for burns on wounded soldiers until he was discharged.

He came home to many changes. My mother had sold the big brick house on Main Street and bought a small two-story white frame house at the north end of Normal at 409 Grant Street in the Wall Glen Addition. The neighborhood had many small two-story houses and a lot of one-story bungalows. She had explained all of this in her letters to Dad and he had been supportive of her decisions at the time, but Dad immediately wanted a larger house.

She had also sold his wooden runabout boat. The local secondhand dealer had convinced her that it would be ruined by dry rot, hanging from the ceiling of the garage, by the time he got home. Dad was sure that the boat was out of the weather and well varnished so it would not have deteriorated.

After the war Dad tried to buy a boat, but used boats were scarce and new boats were not being made yet, because of the material shortages caused by the war. When pleasure boat construction began again, he ordered a boat, but had to wait almost a year for delivery. He still had an old five-horsepower Johnson outboard motor that would still start on the first or second pull. Outboard motors were scarce also.

After the first year of the new boat, the bottom was all scummy from whatever grew in muddy Lake Bloomington so the boat had to be scraped, sanded, and painted. Dad did not have time for this, so Bruce and I sanded and re-sanded the old paint from the bottom until it met his satisfaction. Then we applied a new coat of paint. Antifouling bottom paint was new then, but my father found out about it and got some to paint the boat below the waterline. We put masking tape along the waterline and painted a one-inch-wide red stripe along the waterline to separate the white paint above the water from the copper bottom paint.

After the paint dried, we turned the boat over and filled it with water. The water ran out through the seams between the boards because they had dried out over the winter and shrunk when the boat was covered with a tarp. We had to keep refilling the boat with water until the wood swelled and sealed the leaks.

Dad had a friend who did metalwork. He bent rebar rods to form arches that fit into the oarlocks. These supported the boat cover to keep water from collecting in it.

One of Dad's patients owned a furniture company with a big open bed truck. He agreed to haul the boat to the lake. We knew that the boat did not leak anymore because we had to dump the water out of the boat before loading it onto the truck.

Dad would run the boat around the lake to look at the cabins along the lake and show Bruce and me how to steer the boat. Mom did not swim and hated the boat, so she never went with us. We would beach the boat and walk in the woods that bordered the lake. Dad taught us how to recognize certain trees and how to find morel mushrooms. We found jack-in-the-pulpit flowers and learned to spot poison ivy. There were shaggy bark hickory trees that he pointed out as a source of dry kindling in the forest. Dad taught me how to move around in a boat, run the motor, and do the maneuvers needed to dock the boat when I was seven years old.

When Dad returned from White Sulfur Springs, he had to resume his practice. He arranged for the relocation of the woman who had moved into his old office space and talked the landlord into repairing some damages from neglect so he could use his old office above the town library.

His car had been in storage, so the engine had to be reconditioned and the old tires replaced before he could drive it.

He went to the hospital and found that they had not kept up with medical progress and that the hospital was dirty and run-down. He made it a point to attend the next meeting of the board of directors of Brokaw Hospital. He told the board that they either needed to clean up and modernize the hospital or shut it down. He said that he was embarrassed to bring a patient to that hospital. The board voted to have a fund-raising campaign and, if necessary, sell bonds to raise money to remodel the hospital and add a new surgical wing.

Many citizens of Normal and all the doctors contributed to the effort, and the hospital soon added a new wing. When the doctors discovered that the hospital board had not allowed funds for air-conditioning of the new operating rooms, they got together and donated more money to add the air-conditioning for the operating rooms. They did not want their sweat dripping into surgical openings on hot summer afternoons.

His medical practice kept him very busy. On weekdays, my dad would get up at about 7:00 a.m. and get dressed. Mom would have breakfast on the table by seven thirty so he could leave the house by seven fifty and make it to Brokaw Hospital, one mile away, by eight o'clock for surgery. He would operate one or two cases in the morning and then go to the office in "downtown" Normal to see his postoperative patients. He would come home at noon for lunch and listen to *Paul Harvey News* when he could. Back to the office by one o'clock, he would see office patients until five to six o'clock and eat dinner at home promptly at six o'clock unless he ran late at the office.

The family always ate together. Sometimes he talked about what Bruce and I did in school; sometimes Dad talked to Mom about his patients. Dad was a Truman Democrat and Mom was a Dewey Republican, so we did not discuss politics very much. By seven o'clock, he was back in his car to make house calls. He tried to finish the house calls and get home in time for the ten o'clock news. There was always a stack of current medical journals on the table beside his recliner in the living room. He usually fell asleep during the news and weather while reading journals in his recliner. After the news, Mom would wake him up and tell him to go to bed.

On Saturdays, he made hospital rounds and house calls, trying to finish before lunch. In the afternoon, if he did not have emergencies, he would try to spend time with Bruce and me or work in the garden. Bruce and I were usually drafted to help with the gardening. His favorite flowers were roses. He had a large bed of named rosebushes that he fussed over and liked to show to friends.

He was a very exacting boss. Our jobs were usually to clean up after him and do the "grunt work" of digging and hauling. Mom said that he was accustomed to having nurses come after him to clean up. She thought that he actually did not know how to clean up after himself.

On Sunday mornings, Mom would take us to Sunday school and church. We sat in the back pew in church and saved room for Dad in case he finished his house calls in time for church. Sometimes he would slide into the pew in the middle of the sermon. Dad told me while I was in medical school that he did not believe that anyone could practice medicine very long without acquiring a belief in God. I was reminded of this when a patient gave me a painted barn wood sign that said, "God heals, the doctor takes the fee." He did not make it to church very often when he was in active practice, but became a pillar in the church in Arkansas after he retired.

We would often eat out after church. The Graham's Cafeteria on the courthouse square in Bloomington and the cafeteria at Illinois Wesleyan University were Dad's favorite places. On special occasions, we would go to Streid's on the US 66 beltway where Bruce and I could order any of the bottom-three entrees. They were arranged by price. Sunday afternoons were for family time, again, if Dad did not have emergencies, which occurred quite frequently.

One Saturday afternoon in the summer, the whole family was at home in the little house in the Wall Glen neighborhood. A neighbor came to the door and yelled, "Dr. Barber, come quick! There has been an accident."

Dad went out the door and followed the neighbor who had called for him. Bruce and I went to the door and could see that there was a crowd forming about half a block from our house, but Mom told us to stay at home. The land dropped off between our house and the road below, so we could not see what had happened.

In a few minutes, Dad came back to the house for a box and a small shovel. We asked if we could go to see what happened, but Dad said that we were to stay home and not go near the accident.

We learned later that a little girl had been riding her new bicycle in the street (there were no sidewalks) when a dump truck illegally drove through the neighborhood and passed her. As it passed her, she lost her balance and fell in front of the rear wheels of the dump truck. The truck had crushed her head, killing her instantly.

Being the doctor in the neighborhood, it fell to him to clean up after the accident. He was probably better equipped psychologically to handle the job than anyone else available. He was always willing to accept this kind of responsibility for unpleasant tasks.

As was customary at that time, Brokaw hospital had its own nursing school. The local doctors assisted the nursing faculty in teaching the nursing students. Dad gave lectures once or twice each month and spent time on the hospital floors training the nurses. He was very proud of the nursing graduates and always managed to attend capping and graduation ceremonies each spring. Many of the graduates immediately found jobs at Brokaw Hospital, so he worked with them for years to come.

He also admitted patients to the Mennonite Hospital and St. Joseph's Catholic Hospital in Bloomington. He was always biased toward Brokaw, partly because it was closer to our home so the driving time was less and partly because he had a close relationship with the hospital board. St. Joseph's was way across Bloomington, and he did not like to go there because the Catholic doctors all had first priority for admitting patients and scheduling surgery. He usually had priority at Brokaw for eight o'clock surgery starting time, but had to schedule "to follow" cases at St. Joseph's. "To follow" cases were unpredictable as to when they could be done. He was on a level field with the doctors at Mennonite Hospital.

St. Joseph's was out in southwest Bloomington, near the railroad station. They had the largest ward of iron lung machines, so his polio patients were usually hospitalized at St. Joseph's. Many of Dad's Catholic patients wanted to go to St. Joseph's, so he would accommodate them.

I remember riding with him to St. Joseph's in the evening when he went there to make evening rounds. Bruce and I waited in the car in the parking lot while he made his rounds. In Bloomington and Normal, no one locked their cars; and if it was hot, we rolled down the windows. They were always manual crank windows. Electric windows had not been invented. We never worried about abduction or molestation in those days.

Chapter 10

My father was very unhappy with the new house in the north end of Normal, so he started to plan a new house shortly after he returned from the war. My parents had purchased two lots on Broadway at the south end of Normal during the 1930s. The lots were very close to Brokaw Hospital. Mom and Dad had planned a two-story house of Tudor architecture before the war. We had an architect's model of that house in the storage area, which eventually wound up on my train layout. After the war, they decided they wanted something more modern.

They hired an architect who had worked with Frank Lloyd Wright before moving to Bloomington. Using some of Wright's ideas, he designed a sprawling prairie-style ranch house that spread over the two adjoining lots. The exterior was stone from Lannon, Wisconsin, near Milwaukee. The roof was covered with dark-red flat tiles. The windows were either large pane picture windows with aluminum framing or aluminum casement windows. Double-pane windows were new, but all the windows were double glazed. The summer I was nine years old, I spent many hours watching the workmen as they built the house.

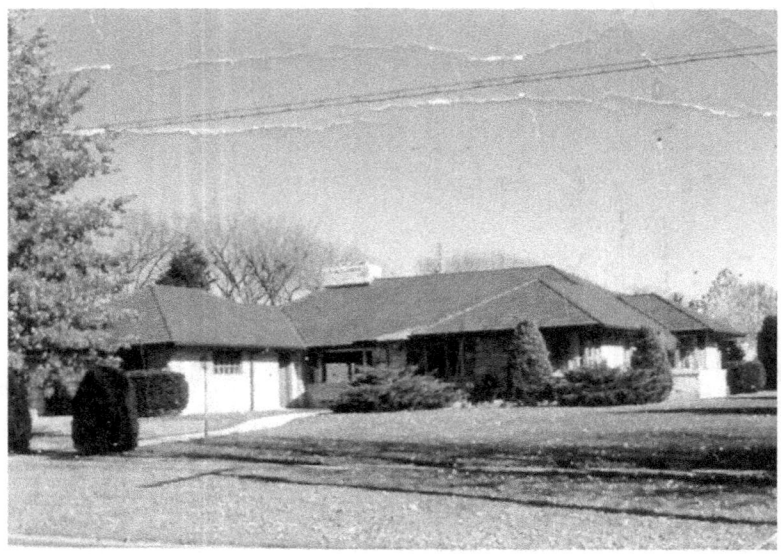

Barber house at 1204 Broadway, Normal, Illinois. Built in 1947–48.

Dad had his basic requirements, but it was Mom's job to plan the details. Dad wanted a one story house with a partial full basement. The exterior had to be as near to maintenance free as possible. Mom wanted a "Pullman Kitchen" and lots of closet space. There was a large L-shaped living and dining room with a black and gold marble shadow box fireplace. The contractor had to call in the marble mason from the cemetery to figure out how to assemble the pre-cut pieces that formed the face of the fireplace.

A den, just inside the front door, was convenient for Dad to see patients when necessary. The house had three bedrooms with a bathroom in the master bedroom suite and another bathroom between the other two bedrooms. There was a powder room between the kitchen and the game room.

When they dug the foundation, we measured the black topsoil. It was six feet deep. Then they hit yellow clay. It took as long to dig the last two feet of clay as it did to dig the black topsoil. The house was shaped like the letter *H* with the garage, kitchen, and game room on one side; the living and dining room and den in the crossbar; and the three bedrooms comprising the other side.

The center of the house had a full basement while the north and south wings had a three-foot-high crawl space connected with the basement. The furnace and hot-water heater were in the basement. Dad told me that the warmth of the furnace heated the crawl space to keep the floors warm in winter. There was open space for a work bench, a deep freezer, washer and dryer, and room for various projects. Shelves along the walls provided storage for hunting and fishing equipment and miscellaneous stuff.

They poured the concrete for the entire main floor in one day so there would not be any discontinuity in the concrete to crack. They started at 5:00 a.m. and finished at 9:00 p.m. on a long midsummer day. The plumbing and electrical conduits were all in the floor before the pour.

Bruce and I both had CO_2-cartridge powered model race cars that ran on a guide wire. The finished concrete floor made a great surface on which to race these cars after the workers left for the day. Unfortunately, in a few days, they started erecting walls around and across the smooth concrete floor, so we could not race the cars at the new house anymore.

The outside walls were made of nine-inch-square red building blocks stacked on their square side. The blocks had three channels. The builders stuffed glass wool insulation in the inner and outer compartments of the tile blocks that made the outside walls. Toward the outside, there was an air space of about one inch between the tiles and the four-inch-thick veneer of random-sized Lannon stone. The outside windowsills consisted of one long piece of Lannon stone while the inside sills were of gray marble. The inside sills were level so Mom could put plants and Christmas decorations in the windows, but Mom regretted the level sills because water condensed on the aluminum window frames and puddled on the sills.

When the stone was delivered in a railroad gondola car, Dad was told that the car would be parked on a siding in Normal for only twenty-four hours until it had to be removed. Bruce and I were enlisted to help unload the stone into trucks to transport it to the building site. I was fascinated to watch the stonemasons break and shape the stone as they laid the walls.

The inside surfaces of the outside walls were covered with insulation board, wire lath, and plaster. The inner walls were made of studs with wire lath and plaster. There was one steel beam that went from one end of the living and dining room space to the other, which was about thirty feet long. The joists and rafters that rested on that beam were wood and were closely spaced to support the heavy red tile roof. The floor in the living and dining rooms was carpeted, but the rest of the house was tiled with either asphalt or cork tiles. They were new and modern—a Frank Lloyd Wright touch.

Years later, when the next owner tried to put in an intercom system, workers had to use jackhammers to run the wiring through the solid concrete floor.

The roofing tiles were special order and my father worried about patching the roof if a tree fell on it, so he ordered more tile than was needed to cover the roof. Bruce and I duck-walked several hundred clay tiles into the three-foot-high crawl space to save them for the future.

The two lots combined were eighty feet deep and one hundred feet wide. On the two lots behind the house, there were a red brick bungalow and an empty lot full of weeds. There was a ten-foot-wide-by-five-foot-high picture window that looked out from the living room into the backyard. My father did not like the view, so he planted specimen evergreen trees all across the backyard to make the red house and vacant lot disappear.

The house was off center on the lot, so there was a wide side yard on the south side. It was wide enough for a badminton or croquet court. My father wanted outdoor lighting but did not want ugly lights on the roof or side of the house, so he designed his own system. The roof had a three-foot overhang past the walls of the house that ran around the whole house. This overhang was to keep rain off the windows and sun off the walls in the summer.

He had boxes built into the eaves with drop-down doors. Floodlights were mounted on the inside of the doors and were connected to mercury switches attached to the doors. When the doors were closed, the switches were horizontal and the lights turned off; but when the doors were open to bring out the lights, the switches were vertical so the lights came on. The lights were on swivels to point wherever the light was needed. There were two of them for the backyard and one for the side yard.

When the concrete was poured for the driveway, they embedded a large coil, which was about a foot wide and four feet long, into the surface. This was connected to the switch for the electric garage door opener. He had the electrician for the house, who was also a ham radio enthusiast, design radio transmitters with coil antennas to mount under the front of his car to activate the garage door opener. This was very new in 1948. People would comment on it when they had driven by and seen the door open when Dad drove into the driveway.

Doctors had to go out in all kinds of weather, so Dad wanted a way to get into the garage without getting out of his car. My mother had an opener for her car so she could also open the heavy double door without getting out of her car to push a button.

Several years later, when my parents visited Florida and became fans of shuffleboard, the coil in the driveway became a local hazard when they painted a shuffleboard court on the driveway. The court was also nonstandard because the driveway was not level. One way was slightly uphill and the other way was downhill.

The house had a large game room. (The term "family room" came later.) It had a multicolored asphalt tile floor and knotty pine paneling that was stained green. There was a deep, narrow cabinet in one corner that could hold the two halves of a folded ping-pong table. It had a top shelf, with a separate flush door with no hardware where they kept the liquor (for parties).

On one wall of the game room was a four-foot-by-eight-foot panel that folded down on hinges with fold-out legs to form a large table. This was for my train layout. We had a neighbor in the Wall Glen Addition who was a model railroader. Dad hired him to come out to the new house to lay an oval of track with switches for a parallel line for two-thirds of the loop. There were built-in shelves in the recess for the table to hold the train cars and locomotives. Unfortunately, there was only about one inch of clearance above the tracks when the table was folded into the wall, so nothing more than an inch high could be built permanently on the tabletop.

My parents could set up half of the ping-pong table in that room, so their group of four couples could play pinochle. We also had duck diners for twenty people or more in that room at the end of duck season, using the two halves of the ping-pong table and card tables.

The hall in the bedroom part of the house had a wall of storage. There were three big closets with double sliding doors. One cabinet had shelves; the other two had hanging bars for out-of-season clothing. Each bedroom had generous closet space. The three closet doors in the master bedroom were covered with floor-to-ceiling mirrors that were hinged to make a three-way mirror when the end closets were opened.

In 1948, the house cost about sixty thousand dollars, making it one of the most expensive houses in the little town of Normal. My father refused to go into debt by taking out a mortgage, so he sold some of his stock portfolio to pay for the house. He was sorry later when his Timken Roller Bearing stock that he had sold had doubled and tripled in value. My mother told him "I told you so" many times, but he was proud to own the house free and clear. She thought he should have used other people's money with a mortgage and kept his stock.

My mother's father had lost most of his money in the crash of 1929 because he had bought stock on margin. I think he influenced my father to never go into debt. My father told me that if I had to borrow money to buy something, I could not afford it. I have not followed that advice when buying houses or cars, but I did pay cash for my Cal 33 sailboat.

The one step at the front door was the only step in the house, except the stairs to the basement. The entrance from the garage was ramped, and the back door was ramped onto the patio. Dad would tell guests that when he and Mom got old, they could wheel themselves in, out, and around the house in their wheelchairs. They planned to retire and stay in Normal.

Chapter 11

Once the house was built and paid for, my father started going to national medical meetings. He went to one in Boston and took my mother along. Casey moved into the house briefly to look after Bruce and me while they were gone.

Casey was dating two men at that time—one during the week and one on weekends. The one on weekends, Art, was an engineer/sales representative for International Harvester who traveled during the week. The other, Ernie, was a wheeler-dealer entrepreneur. Ernie always wanted to get rid of Bruce and me to be alone with Casey. Art wanted to play catch with us or take us hunting. We told Casey to marry Art, which she did. Years later, Casey put her stamp of approval on Judy and Letha before Bruce and I married them.

While Dad went to the meeting in Boston, he sent my mother to the bookstores on Milk Street to find the books on Arctic exploration that he had partially read in Greenland. She managed to find several books by Perry, Bartlett, and other Arctic explorers.

The College of Surgeons had organized a tour to Bermuda following the Boston meeting. My parents went on that tour and thoroughly enjoyed it. When they flew home, my father had an ear infection that left him with a partial loss of the hearing in his left ear from which he never recovered. His hearing was good in his right ear, so he did not wear a hearing aid. He was very afraid that his patients would think he could not hear heart murmurs and breath sounds and therefore might make an error in treatment because of it. He never thought that it hindered him while he practiced medicine.

The trip to Bermuda rekindled his love of travel that he had acquired from his train trips in the army. Two years later, the College of Surgeons organized a trip around South America. It was part cruise, part air, and part train travel. They visited the medical schools of most of the South American countries for lectures and surgical demonstrations. Between meetings, they saw most of South America.

Several years later, the meeting was in Hawaii. They loved the tropical climate and the lush gardens. They had not seen active volcanoes and black sand beaches before. At that time, all tourists in Hawaii traveled by limousine. The drivers were the entertainers at the hotels, so the drivers sang Hawaiian songs and stole fresh pineapples from the fields for the tourists as they drove around the islands. It was very magical.

Shortly after the trip to Hawaii, Mom and Dad celebrated their twenty-fifth wedding anniversary. Dad had princess orchids shipped in from Hawaii for all the women at the party, and everyone was given a lei of yellow Hawaiian plumeria flowers.

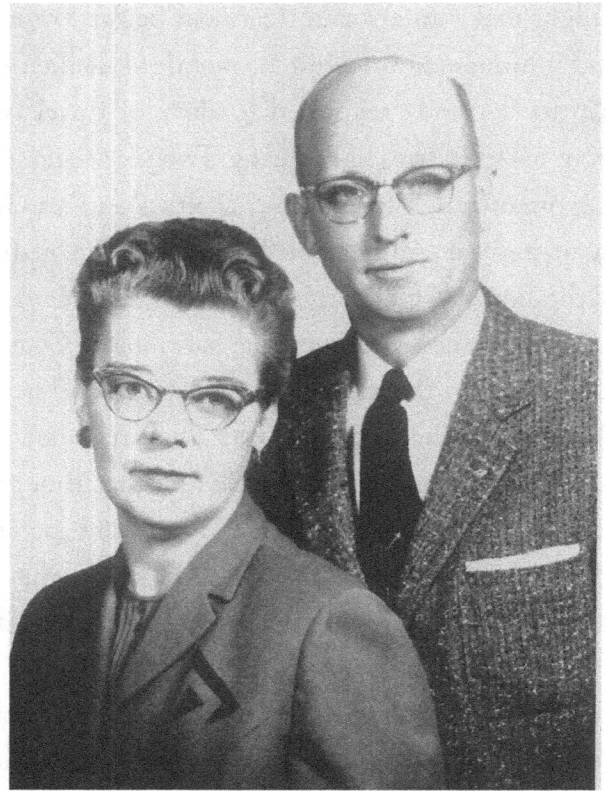

Harry and Edith Barber at their 25th wedding anniversary, February 10, 1959.

One of Dad's hobbies was photography. He took pictures of his flowers and of people, but his main use of his cameras was on vacations. He belonged to a group called the Kodaroamers. This group would get together for a member to show slides of their latest trip. Dad would work for hours selecting his best slides to put together a presentation when it was his turn. Many of these meetings were family picnics, so I saw some of these travelogs.

The group would make an annual trip to the Walgreen estate in northern Illinois to photograph the gardens. Dad loved to take close-up photographs of the flowers. They also went to nearby Starved

Rock, a rocky cliff along the Illinois River in northern Illinois. It got its name from a battle between the Ottawa and the Pottawatomi Indians.

During a council meeting of the Illinois Indians, the chief of the Pottawatomi Indians stabbed the chief of the Ottawa Indians. Fearing reprisals, the Pottawatomi Indians took refuge on the high, easily defended rock. The Ottawa Indians trapped them there, and the Pottawatomies eventually died of starvation. It is now the most visited park in Illinois. Dad was so impressed by the story that he took Bruce and me there to see the rock.

I remember seeing movies at one of these meetings made by a naturalist, showing a squirrel entering a milk bottle containing several nuts. The squirrel put the nuts in his mouth and then could not get out of the bottle because his head full of nuts was too big for the neck of the bottle. He would not spit out the nuts, so they had to break the bottle for the squirrel to escape. Dad let us know that he thought it was immoral to treat animals in this way.

One of the members had a hobby of taking black-and-white photographs of flowers and then hand painting them with watercolors, using fine brushes under high magnification. I was really impressed, having tried to paint model train cars by hand. In my teaching career, I often hand painted my text slides to give them color and make them stand out, but that was gross work compared to painting the flowers.

Photography was about the only hobby other than gardening that Dad had time for, and that was mostly on vacation and several evenings afterward to arrange his slides. He took it very seriously and was always concerned about composition, lighting, and proper exposures. He would get upset if his cameras leaked light and cause his pictures to be "light struck." Sometimes he could mask out the light-struck parts with silver tape to save an otherwise good picture. He took great pride in a well-composed and well-exposed photograph.

Chapter 12

After the war, Dad started going on fishing trips to Wisconsin or Minnesota, usually with a group of men. They would fish for walleye, bass, northern pike, and muskie. On one trip to Wisconsin, he hooked a muskie and fought it for about thirty minutes before getting it along the side of the boat. The guide tried to gaff the muskie to get it into the boat, but he missed! The muskie made a big lunge and broke the line. That was the closest Dad ever got to catching a muskie, although he kept trying.

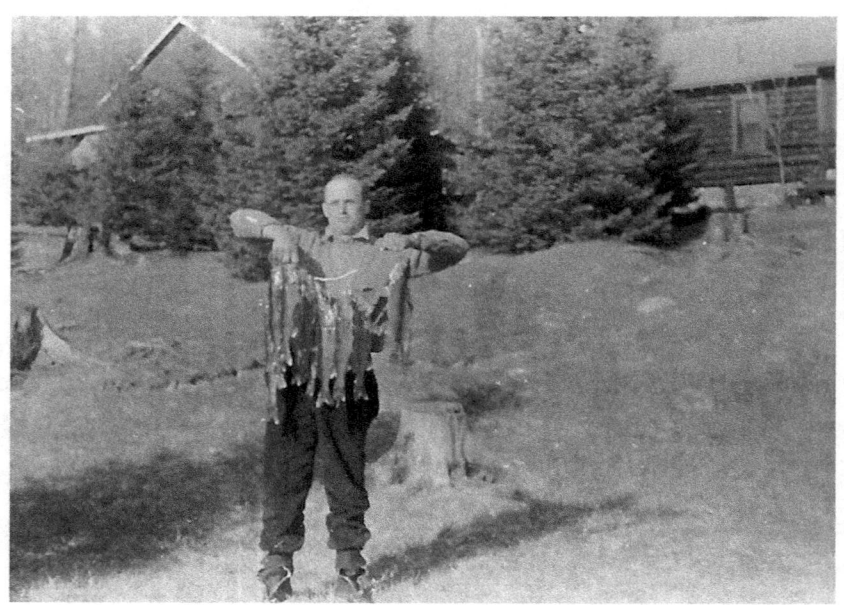

Caption: Harry Barber holding a string of walleyed pike caught in Minnesota about 1948.

One summer, my mom and dad went fishing with their best friends, Lee and Mary Alice Long. Mary Alice always went by the nickname "Sugar." They drove to the end of the Gunflint Trail in Minnesota and rented a cabin. After two days of fishing, they had to skip a day of fishing to go into town for groceries. This meant forty miles each way on a dusty washboard dirt road.

Mom and Sugar shopped while Dad and Lee walked around the little town. After shopping, they drove back the forty miles of dusty washboard road. Two days later, they had run out of groceries and had to go back to town. The women had bought only one head of lettuce and a few other items of food. The men accused the women of deliberately buying only two day's supplies so they could go back to town rather than fishing. That was the last time the women went along.

Dad loved the western United States. He had seen parts of it from the back platforms of troop trains, but he wanted to go back to experience the mountains, lakes, and wildlife. We started to take vacation trips to the west, when I was about nine years old. We would start at sunrise and head north, up US 51, to LaSalle where we picked up US 6 going west. One year, we followed US 6 to Denver to see Colorado. Dad loved to keep the speedometer needle pointed straight up at sixty miles per hour, a mile a minute.

Going across rolling Iowa was like riding a roller coaster, but straight. We sped up one side of a hill and down the other side. When we got to Kansas, it was flat. As we past one alfalfa drier, we could see the next one, several miles down the road. The smell of drying alfalfa was continuous from one elevator to the next. Huge combines swept across the wheat fields in groups of three. The highways were always two lanes, so we had to pass frequently to maintain the sixty miles per hour. Dad was very good at estimating the time it would take him to pass another car before the oncoming car arrived.

There were no interstates, so we went through all the small towns. We would stop at the corner restaurant in the center of some small town for lunch and stay in a roadside motel at night. We did not have reservations so we had to stop before the motels filled up.

Dad had an aversion to staying at fancy motels with swimming pools or playgrounds. He said that they were more expensive because of the extras and we were only there to sleep. His background of growing up poor and living through the Depression stayed with him.

Another year, we followed US 34 to Cheyenne, Wyoming. We met the Longs there and went to the Cheyenne Stampede. That was our first rodeo and the contestants were real working cowboys. The Longs were driving Mom's Chevy coupe because Lee had a company car that he could not drive for personal use. The little 1940 Chevy climbed Pikes Peak after they left us to see Colorado.

We went west to the Tetons and Yellowstone. My brother was always getting carsick and the sulfur smell of Yellowstone made it worse, so we did not stay there very long. Dad had a way of driving that I thought was conducive to carsickness. He would accelerate for a few seconds and then coast until the car started to decelerate. Then he would push the gas pedal to accelerate again. He said that this saved gas. People have told me that this makes them carsick. When Bruce sat in the front seat, he could look out of the windows at the horizon, which is one of the suggested cures for seasickness. Mom would sit in the back with me, but I never got to sit up front because I never got carsick.

We went north through Glacier National Park and into Canada, but did not do the "Going to the Sun Highway." We stayed one night at Lake Louise and continued driving north to see the Athabasca

Glacier before turning around and heading home. Dad gave us a long lecture on glaciers and moraines while we walked on the glacier. He told us about the glaciers in Greenland again. We returned through Montana to see the big open pit copper mines and watch them refine copper and make copper wire.

Dad was always concerned about the car breaking down on these trips. He checked the oil at every gasoline stop and decided on one trip when we were in Portland, Oregon, that it was time to have the oil changed. There was a filling station across the street from our motel, so he took the car over for an oil change. The next morning, we drove to the coast and started south down the Pacific coastal highway. The car started running rough. The farther we went, the rougher the engine ran. By the time we made it to Coos Bay, Dad decided to get it checked. It was almost noon on Saturday, so he was afraid that the repair shops would close. We were lucky to find a Buick dealer who was open. Dad had a mechanic check the car.

The mechanic discovered that several of the valves were stuck and that two of the valves were stuck in the open position. The pistons had repeatedly hit the open valves because the stuck valves were extended into the cylinders. This bent the valves until they would not seat. To repair the car, they had to pull the head off the engine; clean the valves, replace the bent ones, and reassemble the engine before replacing the oil. They told Dad that the filling station had used high detergent oil, which had freed up all the accumulated gunk in the engine, gumming up the valve lifters.

Dad never met a stranger and could talk with anyone. He convinced the mechanic that we needed the car repaired as fast as possible, so the mechanic worked all Saturday afternoon and Sunday morning to get the car fixed. We stayed in a motel near the garage, so we did not see much of Coos Bay. They delivered the car at noon on

Sunday, so we made it into California Sunday night and saw Crater Lake the next day.

Dad hated to drive in big cities, so we did not go to San Francisco but went to Sacramento and over the mountains, through Donner Pass, to Reno, and then back home to Illinois. Dad told us the story of the Donner party being stranded in a mountain pass and dying of starvation. He taught us about the immorality of cannibalism.

Every spring, we would have an Easter break from school. It started on Palm Sunday and went through Easter. In about 1950, we started going to Florida for that week. The first year, we flew to from Chicago to Tampa where we met Granddad Bentzen for lunch at the Vinoy Hotel in central St. Petersburg. Granddad was upset by the number of young blond women who were disgracefully chasing old widowers. Since he was a wealthy widower, Mom was worried that one might catch him.

We drove south to Naples and spent several days on the beach there before going to Miami Beach. Dad would not stay in Miami Beach—it was too expensive—so we drove north to Hollywood. The motels there were only on the beach side of the road, so we got to stay on the beach. The restaurant next to the motel had a sign in the window that they took Diners Club cards. Credit cards were new. Dad asked about them at the restaurant and decided he had to have one. He usually traveled with a lot of cash and a letter of credit from the bank at home in case he needed money for an emergency. With the letter, the local bank would take his check for cash. He liked the idea of charging everything to a credit card rather than carrying large amounts of cash.

We walked on the beach with Dad while he pointed out starfish, sand dollars, and several types of shells. He found a bluish purple balloon on the beach and picked it up to look at it closely. He immediately dropped it and began shaking his hand. The balloon had stung him. A man came over to tell Dad that he had just picked up a Portuguese man-of-war. We examined several of these that had washed up on the beach but did not touch them. They had tentacles about three feet long that hung down in the water and stung anything they contacted.

The next year, we drove our car to Florida and made it to Tupelo, Mississippi, the first night. Mom saw signs along the road for a motel in Tupelo that was "Modern as Tomorrow." Dad wanted to stop when it got dark, but she insisted on staying at the "modern" motel in Tupelo and urged that Dad drive on. When we arrived in Tupelo, the motel was full and there were no vacancies nearby. They put us in a room in a house behind the motel that had linoleum floors and a sink and commode that dated back to World War I or before. After that experience, whenever we stayed in a motel that was not up to par, Dad would say it was "Modern as Tomorrow."

We ate lunch with one of Dad's army friends from Greenland in Mobile, Alabama, on the way to Apalachicola, Florida. Dad wanted some of the fresh shrimp that the Florida coast was famous for, so we went to a drive-in that featured fried shrimp. We all had fried shrimp baskets. About an hour later, I broke out in hives all over. Dad was allergic to oysters, so he thought I was allergic to shellfish. Dad told me not to eat either shrimp or oysters after that. By the time I was in college, I was eating both without any reaction.

We drove on the next day to Clearwater Beach. Dad thought the beach hotels there were too fancy and too expensive, so we drove south to Indian Rocks Beach. Dad refused to stay at a motel on the beach side of the road because they were too expensive. He found one across the road, and we stayed there for several days. We could walk through the motel on the beach side of the road to get to the beach.

We tried surf fishing at the beach. I caught a flounder and dragged it up onto the beach. I thought, at first, that it was some kind of trash that I had hooked on the bottom. Dad inspected it, but could not recognize it since it had both eyes on one side and was speckled brown on one side and snow white on the other. A man walking on the beach told us it was a flounder. Dad had never seen a flounder and it was ugly, so I threw it back in the gulf.

We walked down a road that led to the inter-coastal waterway at the back side of the island. A young man there had a little sailboat that he had made from plans in *Popular Mechanics* magazine. It had a closed flat-decked hull about fourteen feet long and three feet wide holding a mast with a triangular sail between two booms called a lateen sail. It had a dagger-board in the center and a rudder attached to the stern. He could sail it around the bay behind the island, and it looked like fun.

Dad was talking to him about the boat and mentioned that he was a doctor. Morris, the man with the boat, told my dad that his father was dying of cancer, but he was upset with his doctor. The doctor would not tell him what to expect from the cancer or how long he might live. Morris asked Dad to go to his house and talk with his father. Dad visited with Morris's dad and explained his cancer to him.

Morris was very pleased that Dad had done this and offered to pay Dad for his time. Dad told him that he was on vacation, so he would not accept money, but it would be nice if Morris would teach Bruce and me how to sail his boat. We had several sessions with Morris over the next few days, and Bruce and I began a lifelong love of sailing. This homemade boat was the precursor to the sailfish and sunfish sailboats that are seen all over the world today. Dad did not like sailing because you had to tack to go upwind. He wanted to point the bow at the destination, rev the motor, and go.

A storm passed through the area while we were there, leaving a lot of sponges on the beach. I collected some of the sponges, and Dad found a book on sponges in one of the gift shops. We decided that my science project that year would be about sponges. I kept the sponges on some newspapers next to the door of our room to dry. When it was time to go home, the sponges started to smell really bad, so Dad would not let me put them in the trunk of the car. I left them behind and changed the science project to the seashells I had collected on the beach instead. Bruce used the book on sponges as the basis of his science project, but without the smelly sponges.

Chapter 13

After the war, we started visiting my father's family in Richmond, Missouri, during the summer. We would go for a long weekend. My grandfather was still living, but my grandmother Barber died when I was a year old. Dad had two brothers who were still alive—Olin and Frank.

Olin lived on a farm a few miles out of Richmond that Dad had bought for him. He had served in World War II and been discharged because of heart problems. He was on medical disability and had Veterans Administration health coverage. He took the disability label to extremes and decided it meant that he should not ever try to work again.

Olin was married to Lucille and had two sons, Raymond and Dorris. Both boys were in high school when we started to visit them. My father supported Olin, in addition to his disability check, to keep his family in food and housing. Dad bought a forty-acre farm near Richmond and moved them onto it. Dad hoped that they could raise vegetables and chickens so they could partially live off the land.

Lucille and Olin had married right after high school graduation. She was the daughter of the local judge, and everyone thought they had everything going for them. They went on a joy ride for their honeymoon in the new car the judge gave them as a wedding present. They rode around the west until they ran out of money and had to come home. Olin did various jobs until he was drafted for World War

II. After the war, he claimed that he could not work because of his "heart trouble" and became an alcoholic.

The first time we visited them, Olin was sitting under a tree in front of the house, holding a bottle of whiskey. Lucille and the boys were in the house. We went into the house and sat on some old couches while Dad asked Lucille what she needed for food and maintenance of the house. He made a list of food and other things they needed.

Each year when we visited, we would go to the farm to evaluate things and then go to town to buy sacks of flour and sugar and order a drum of kerosene to be delivered to the farm for the kerosene cooking stove and oil lamps. Dad would make arrangements for heating oil and arrange credit for Lucille at the grocery store. Dad would send checks to Lucille, but Olin would intercept the mail and cash the checks to keep the money to buy booze.

There was a well with a hand pump near the kitchen door, but no plumbing in the house. The farm was my first experience with the Sears catalog in the outhouse. (We had outhouses at Camp Manitou, but they had toilet paper.) They did not have electricity at the farm. Cooking was done on a coal oil stove; lighting was by kerosene lanterns.

We always had a bad case of fleas after visiting the farm. Dad had to get flea spray to spray us and our clothes to be rid of the fleas. We stayed in the hotel in Richmond once, but it was grim, so after that, we stayed at the Oaks Hotel in Excelsior Springs. The white sheets at the hotel brought out the fleas. We looked like we had measles for several days because of the flea bites.

Dad would buy a sow for them and have it bred so they could raise hogs for food and income. The price of the breeding at another farm was usually a pick of the litter once the pigs were born. Dad learned that as soon as the pigs were weaned, Olin had the sow butchered for food and asked Dad to buy him another sow. As soon as the pigs were partially grown, Olin had them slaughtered for food. That ended the effort at making Olin more self-sufficient as a pig farmer.

The oldest son, Raymond, was a good student and had real promise. His senior year in high school, he started working for several local farmers. He knew how to drive a tractor to plow and plant crops, so he made enough money to support the family. The night he graduated from high school, he and a buddy bought a case of Coca-Cola and decided to drink it that night all by themselves. Raymond passed out, so he was taken unconscious to the hospital emergency room where he died.

Dad learned from the emergency room doctor that Raymond had died in diabetic acidosis before they determined what was wrong. Dad was looking forward to Raymond supporting the family, relieving him of the responsibility.

Dorris was two years younger and did not do better than average in school. After graduation from high school, he got a job in a junkyard cutting up auto bodies with a torch for scrap. The story I heard was that he made the owner's daughter pregnant in the backseat of a junked car while working there, so he lost that job.

Shortly after that, he married a nurse who worked at a hotel in Excelsior Springs, Missouri. She got him a job as an orderly at the hotel that specialized in spring-water bath treatments for various ailments. Each room had a list of diseases with the prices of the baths for each under the glass top on the dresser. Dorris would transport the guest to and from the baths by wheelchair or gurney. This marriage and job ended when he wrecked his car while he was with another woman while his wife was at work.

A friend got him a job at the Firestone tire plant in Kansas City. The workers would be picked up every morning by the company bus and delivered back to the stop every evening. Dorris decided that he did not like to work more than two weeks straight, so he soon lost that job. He went through several jobs before settling down and marrying the other woman. We never learned much about her except that she chewed tobacco and had a teenage daughter from a previous marriage.

Olin died a few years after Dorris graduated from high school. Olin's wife, Lucille, lived in town for several years before dying from complications of diabetes. Dad had sold the farm after Olin died, so she lived in an apartment in town on welfare and disability and support from Dorris and Dad.

Every few years, Dorris would call Dad to ask him to cosign a note for Dorris to buy a new car. Dorris always got the top-of-the-line Chevrolet Impala, so Dad grumbled that Dorris was driving a car that was better than his, but had to have a cosigner for his loans. Dad never had to pay for a default on any of the cars. He felt he owed it to his dead brother to look after his family. He often sent money to Lucille after Olin died.

Dad's brother Frank was in the war also. Before the war, he had worked for the Atchison, Topeka, and Santa Fe railroad. After the war, he went back to the railroad. He and his wife Minnie lived on a small farm outside of Topeka and raised chickens and sold eggs for extra income. Minnie's nickname was Aunt Minnie Feedbags because she made underwear and kitchen curtains out of the used chicken feed sacks. She and Frank lived comfortably in the old farmhouse.

Frank worked the mail cars on the trains although he was qualified as a fireman. The mail car paid much better and had better hours. All the brothers had grown up on a farm, so farming was natural for Frank.

Both of Frank's sons, Bob and Frank Jr., inherited muscular dystrophy from Minnie's side of the family. Both had served in World War II and had veteran's benefits. Both were married, but did not have children. They both died of complications of muscular dystrophy in their forties.

Shortly after our new house was built, we visited Richmond again. My grandfather was almost ninety years old and in failing mental health. He lived in a room in a nice boardinghouse in Richmond and spent his days sitting with his friends on the wall of the sidewalk in front of the courthouse, weather permitting. We would find him there when we arrived in town.

Dad wanted him to see the new house to see how far his son had come in the world. We brought Granddad Barber home with us. Granddad thought Dad was foolish to put money into such a fancy house and told him so.

Granddad was supposed to stay for a week until Dad could take him home. I moved in with Bruce because he had a double bed. I turned my room with a single bed over to Granddad. He got confused at night and decided to urinate in the corner of my room. Because of his disorientation and confusion and being in a different house, he was hard for my mother to manage.

Dad was too busy to take time off midweek to take him home, so it was decided to have Bruce take him home to Richmond by Greyhound Bus. This involved changes of buses in St. Louis and Chillicothe, Missouri. Bruce had a terrible time keeping Granddad from boarding the wrong buses at the stopovers, but managed to get him home. Granddad Barber died about a year later at the age of ninety.

Chapter 14

Dad liked to hunt and fish. He grew up in the river bottoms of the Missouri River and took every chance to get back to nature with a fishing rod or a gun. He tried to instill his love of the woods and water into Bruce and me.

When I was seven years old, Dad sent Bruce to Camp Manitou on the shores of the Georgian Bay of Lake Huron. This camp was owned and managed by a group of athletic coaches from Bloomington High School, Illinois State Normal University, and Butler University in Indianapolis. They hired college athletes from the two colleges to serve as counselors and the kitchen staff from the schools to run the commissary.

The camp ran for two months, and campers could sign up for one or both months. Bruce went for the whole time that camp was open. The camp had many canoes, several motorboats, and a big launch. There were about fifteen cabins with eight or nine boys and a counselor in each cabin. There was a big lodge with a recreation room, a dining hall, a nurse's office, and the camp administrative offices.

Older boys went on "Long Lake Trip" in the two-man canoes and packed everything they needed for two weeks of camping and canoeing. The trip followed a string of lakes into the wilderness for fifty miles before turning back and retracing their route. This involved several portages that varied from hundred-foot lift-overs to half-mile hikes through the woods. Since they carried everything they needed, it usually involved at least two trips on each portage for the canoes and equipment. Younger boys went on a separate "Short Lake Trip," which took the route of the first half of "Long Lake Trip" to qualify for either trip; a boy must have been in camp the year before.

Mom and Dad decided that I should go to Camp Manitou when I turned eight. Minimum age for the camp was eight years old. The second term of camp started on the weekend of July 4. Bruce went at the start of camp, so he was already there. Dad took me to camp in his Buick. The two of us went up through Michigan and crossed into Canada at Sault Sainte Marie. Dad took me down to the locks connecting Lake Superior and Lake Huron. He explained how they lifted or lowered the big ore ships from one lake to the next. We watched several ships go through the locks.

To get to camp, we had to go to the little town of Birch Island on the northeast shore of the Georgian Bay. The town had a train station, a general store, a church, a boat landing, and several houses. The launch from the camp met us at the landing to take us across the "thousand islands" part of Georgian Bay to the camp. When we arrived in camp, Dad was told that I could not be in camp until I was eight years old. My birthday was July 12, so I was not supposed to be there yet. I do not recall the reason, but it was probably insurance restrictions.

Dad had brought a two-man arctic survival tent and two sleeping bags (one for my bunk at camp and one for him) and extra camping clothes. He borrowed a motorboat and a canoe from the camp and purchased provisions for camping from the mess hall. Dad talked with people at the camp to learn what nearby islands on the local map of Georgian Bay were used for camping. He took Bruce and me for a five-day camping trip on the islands.

Dad and Bruce and I went into the islands and found a nice island for a camp site. We pitched our tent, built a fireplace with rocks, and gathered firewood. We soon had a comfortable camp. Our days were spent fishing from the canoe around various islands and swimming in the little bay near the campsite. Dad turned out to be a good cook with flour, bacon, canned goods, and the fish we caught.

I caught a good-sized northern Pike and fell over backward in the canoe trying to land it, but did not tip the canoe over. Dad never let me forget my first big fish. We explored several islands and found one that was covered with blueberry bushes. We picked enough berries to fill a gallon can, so Dad fixed blueberry pancakes for breakfast after that.

Bruce and I would paddle the canoe around the little bay and practice getting in and out of it without tipping it over. One day, we followed a deer as it swam from one island to another.

The sleeping arrangements left something to be desired. The floor of our tent was about seven feet long and five feet wide. Dad and Bruce slept side by side in the long direction of the tent. My sleeping bag was crossways at the foot of the tent. Bruce was short enough that his feet did not reach me, but Dad was six feet tall so he kicked me every time he moved. I am sure I did the same to him.

When we returned to Camp Manitou, I was assigned to the cabin with the youngest boys. This was several cabins away from Bruce's cabin, which suited him just fine. They put Dad up in the lodge. He treated several of the boys for minor ailments while he was there.

The young boys were called the Jolly Rogers and did different activities from the rest of the camp. The first day I was there, we climbed the five-hundred-foot-high glacier scarred rock mountain behind the camp to replace the flags on the pole on top of the mountain.

The counselors produced gallon cans with wire bails for us to use to pick blueberries on the way back to camp. Dad was still at camp and met us coming back to camp. He had his own gallon bucket and insisted that I stay to help him fill it when the other boys got tired of picking and went back to camp. He took the bucket of blueberries to Sid's house and talked Sid's wife into baking a blueberry pie for him. (Sid was the caretaker for the camp and lived there with his wife all year round.)

That night, Dad came to get Bruce and me just before Taps and took us up to Sid's house. We drank hot tea and ate warm blueberry pie until about a half hour after Taps. Bruce and I had to sneak back into our cabins. Bruce got away with it, but I got caught by the counselor. I think I got demerits for being out after Taps. My counselor did not care if my dad was in camp—we were supposed to be in the cabin by Taps.

Another night, Dad took Bruce and me with four of the counselors to a shallow grassy bay where we caught over a hundred bullhead catfish in about three hours. That night, I had prior approval to be out late. Several of the counselors spent the next morning skinning and cleaning the catfish so the whole camp could have a catfish dinner. Dad left the next day to drive back to Normal.

A week later, when the big boys went on "Long Lake Trip," one of the boys had an attack of acute appendicitis when he was at the far end of the trip. Coach Howard Saar, who was athletic director for Bloomington High School, part owner of the camp and longtime friend of my father, carried the boy and all of their gear across the portages before going back for the canoe and the remaining gear at each portage. About halfway back the flowage, they reached a logging camp that had shortwave radio to arrange for a pontoon plane to fly to the logging camp lake. The plane took the boy to the hospital in Little Current, Ontario. By the time he arrived in Little Current, his parents had been contacted and they had given permission for surgery. The boy had an appendectomy, survived the appendicitis, and went home to Indiana after his hospital stay.

The next spring, Bruce and I both had our appendixes removed before Dad would let us go back to camp. He had done several emergency appendectomies on soldiers stationed in remote places while he was in the army. He knew of people who had died from appendicitis because they were too far from medical care. Dr. Irwin did the surgery and probably did not get into trouble in those days for removing a normal appendix. Today, a surgeon would get in trouble with the hospital tissue committee if he removed a normal appendix.

Bruce and I went back to Camp Manitou for the whole term the next year, but Dad did not go along. This time, we went by train. We took the GM&O train to Chicago where we had to change train stations to get the train to Toronto. We changed trains again to get to Sudbury. There we caught a local train that stopped at crossroads and little towns until we arrived at Birch Island. There were so many boys that the launch had to tow two war canoes to get us all to camp. Bruce made the Short Lake Trip that year, but I never made a lake trip.

That summer, a group of men from Normal went fishing on Rainy Lake in southern Ontario. Dad heard all about the trip when they returned and decided he wanted to take us there. The next summer, we went by train on the Milwaukee Route, up the Mississippi to Minneapolis/St. Paul. There, we caught what my father called the Toonerville Trolley through the woods of Minnesota to International

Falls. We stopped several times at road crossings for berry pickers and bicyclists to board the train.

A man from Lloyd's Outfitters met us at the train and got us through customs into Fort Francis, Ontario. They put us on a launch along with supplies for the camp and took us thirty-five miles up Rainy Lake to the extreme north end of the lake where a fifty-five-foot cascade tumbles into the lake, creating a huge eddy.

There were two fishing lodges there. One had white clapboard cottages with running water and electricity; the other had log cabins with wood-burning heating stoves, no electricity, and running water that was only available at the dining hall/lodge. We stayed at the log cabins and lit fires in the stoves at six every morning to take the chill off the cabin. Dad taught us to put the wood in the stove at night and splashed kerosene on it, so the fire was easy to light. The Indian boys delivered a pitcher of water to the steps of the cabin every morning before sunrise. Dad said that the warm wool blankets with the six black stripes at one corner were Hudson Bay Blankets. They kept the cold out very well. I wanted one to take home.

One of the supply boxes in the boat was a case of Old Granddad whiskey. Herb, the owner of the lodge, met us on the dock with a wheelbarrow. As soon as he had us headed toward our cabin, he loaded the case of Old Granddad onto his wheelbarrow and headed up the hill toward the lodge. When we came back for the second load of gear to take to the cabin, Herb was halfway up the hill, sitting on the front of the wheelbarrow. He had opened the case and was drinking from the first bottle. We soon learned that Herb had a drinking problem, but had been sober for two weeks since he had run out of whiskey. Herb's daughter, Bea, and son-in-law, Howard, actually ran the camp.

Dad had learned about some good fishing spots from the men in Normal, so he took us in a boat without a guide for a couple of days. There was a bay with several shoals about three miles down the lake and another large rock that was just above the surface of the lake about a half mile from camp. This rock was called John's Rock because John Watchinski from Normal caught about a dozen fish while casting from the rock the year before. He was not feeling well that day, so he had his party put him on the rock while they went down the lake to fish. He caught the most fish in his party that day. We caught some fish at these two places, but not as many as Dad was expecting.

He did get the opportunity to show us again how well he could tie knots without a left thumb. He had a powerful grip between his left index and middle fingers. He showed us one- and two-handed knots and how he could hold and use a hemostat with his left hand. He taught us how to use a hemostat to remove fishhooks from the mouth of the fish. This kept the hooks out of our fingers when the fish shook its head.

Dad was not familiar with the rocks and shoals of Rainy Lake. As a consequence, we hit a shoal with the motor and suddenly we were without any propulsion. Dad pulled the motor into the boat and quickly determined that the shear pin was broken. He always carried a spare pin in his tackle box and proceeded to show Bruce and me how to change a shear pin. He also showed us the spare magneto that he always carried in case the one on the motor went bad.

Dad was not satisfied with our fishing in Rainy Lake, so he hired a guide to take us to good fishing for walleye pike. This involved a portage of about one hundred yards with about thirty feet of elevation change around a waterfall. We towed two canoes for about six miles down Rainy Lake to where a small river entered the east side of the lake. We followed the river for about two miles to the waterfall. The Indian guide carried the canoes across the portage while we carried the other gear.

This took us to Vein Lake and Strong Lake where our guide knew about underwater ridges, which were teeming with walleyes. We caught our limits by lunchtime, ate several for our shore lunch, and went back for more fish to fill our limits again. We fished these lakes for three days and caught the limit of walleyes that we could take out of Canada to ship home. The fish were packed in ice in the log icehouse. Every winter, Herb sawed ice blocks from the lake and stacked them in sawdust in the icehouse where they stayed all summer.

On the third day fishing for walleye pike, our canoe drifted away from the ridge, and I thought I had snagged something on the bottom. My snag eventually became a thirty-six-inch northern pike. Dad said that northern pike were not good to eat because they had too many bones so I should not keep it. When we were about to throw it back, the guide said he would take it to feed to his family. When we returned to Normal, Mom gave Dad a rough time for not bringing it home to be mounted. Dad called northern pike "snakes" because small ones were so thin and were slimy to touch.

Once we had our limits of walleye, we had to find another type of fish to catch. Dad talked with Howard about fishing for bass. Howard knew of a lake that was known for bass. It required a ride up the river above the camp and a short lift-over portage into the midpoint of Sphene Lake, also known as Six Mile Lake. We beached our boat at the west end of Sphene Lake and loaded up our gear for a three-quarter-mile walk through the woods to Elbow Lake. The guide carried a canoe, Dad carried the paddles and lunch, while Bruce and I carried the rest of the gear. Fortunately, there was an old abandoned logging road that covered about half of the distance. We launched the canoe and alternated fishing with two people in the canoe and two on shore.

This lake had several active beaver lodges and many pine trees that the beavers had felled into the lake. Dad taught us to use big splashy plugs that we cast near the fallen trees. The water would explode with a fish hitting the lure as soon as it landed. We had adrenaline-pumping excitement as the bass would fight on the surface with jumps and flips. More than one managed to throw the plug back at us.

The lake had so many trees that the beavers had chewed and pushed into the water that the tannins from the trees gave a golden color to the water and the fish. We caught our limits and had a fish fry lunch to boot.

The guide made the best coffee by boiling lake water in a gallon can, dumping the coffee into the boiling water, and then setting the can aside for the grounds to settle. The fish fillets were shaken with a special breading mixture in a paper bag and deep-fried in bacon grease. I have never had fresher- or better-tasting fish. We quit fishing in time to walk back to our boat on Sphene Lake and make it back to camp before dark.

We repeated the trip again the next day with a second canoe so we could all fish from canoes. Howard decided to leave two canoes at Elbow Lake for other parties to fish there without the hassle of carrying canoes back and forth. We fished that lake for three days and caught all the bass we could take home.

The second day at Elbow Lake, we cooked lunch on a rocky point on the shore of the lake. Dad found a note tacked to the tree that said that three fishermen were waiting for a pontoon plane to pick them up about a week before, so we were not the first to fish that lake that year.

Dad was always willing to help. While we were at Pioneer Lodge the second year, several large parties arrived. This overextended the lodge's supply of boats and motors. The lodge next door was full also. Howard decided to go to Shapiro's Lodge up on Sphene Lake to borrow two canoes and motors. He planned to make the trip by canoe, but needed someone to help paddle. Herb was still on a bender with the fresh supply of bourbon, so Dad volunteered to go with Howard.

After dinner, they paddled to the portage, lifted over, and continued to the upper end of Sphene Lake. They sat and drank coffee all evening because it took Howard until ten o'clock that night to convince Mr. Shapiro that he could lend them two canoes and two motors. They put the motors in the bottom of the canoes to make them easier to tow and set off for our camp.

They were gliding effortlessly along as they approached the portage when the water next to the canoe exploded. Dad was heavier than Howard, so he was in the stern of the canoe. Suddenly, he was eye to eye with a huge moose. The moose had been submerged eating moss off the bottom of the lake when the canoe startled it. It was apparently as surprised as Dad and Howard, so it bolted away. Once they realized that no harm had been done, they had a great laugh. Dad told that story many times.

Dad always took his first aid kit when he went fishing. It had several sterile hemostats, a scalpel, some suture material, a needle holder, some antibiotics, and a sterile end-cutting pliers. Several times, he gave people shots of penicillin. He removed a fishhook from the eyebrow of an Indian boy who was trying to cast a fishing lure when it caught his eyebrow. Dad showed me how to advance the hook until the barb is through the wound and then cut off the tip of the hook with the barb. Then the hook can be pulled back through the tissue without any further damage. He gave the boy a shot of antibiotics, which seemed to hurt him more than the fishhook.

Dad looked on the Indians as poor and undereducated but humans deserving of care and compassion like everyone else. Dad was not a racist, but he had been raised in rural Missouri during segregation and used terms that would be considered racist today. He called black children "picaninnies" and black men who misbehaved, "niggers." He had several black friends from his medical school days for whom he had great respect.

When I grew up in Normal, there was only one black family. The husband ran a barbershop that was frequented by many of the local population. His wife sang in the Presbyterian Church choir. She wore a two-inch riser on one shoe to compensate for the polio she had as a child. She entered the choir loft from the side door rather than process with the choir because of it. They were both Dad's patients. By the time I was in high school, we had four or five black kids in school.

There was a synagogue in Bloomington, but Bruce and I did not know any Jewish people. I did not know much about the Jewish people and certainly could not recognize a Jewish person if I saw one although I was told that they had a certain look. In medical school, I had many Jewish friends. Most did not "look Jewish." Dad did not seem to like Jews and sometimes referred to them as "kikes" and "misers" and associated them with hording money and cheating. This was not unusual among men his age in Bloomington–Normal.

We went back to Pioneer Lodge for three summers. One year when we were there, we noticed that one of the bays on the east side of Rainy Lake was choked with swamp grass. Herb was sober that year. He told us that the grass broke loose from a swamp and became a floating island when the ice went out of the lake. It had drifted down the lake until it was blown into the shallow bay. It took root there and was blocking the access to several houses along the bay. Mando, the paper pulp company, had several large tugboats on the lake to drag log booms to the paper mill in Fort Francis. One of the tugs, along with several big motorboats, tried to tow the floating island out of the bay, but they could not budge it.

Dad went with Herb in the old launch from the lodge called the *Daisy Mae*. It had a motor that sounded like an old John Deere tractor. It would go *putt, putt, putt, pow, putt, putt, putt, pow* as it went down the lake. They nosed the bow of the launch into the island at an angle and revved the motor to rotate the island until the roots broke free a few at a time from the outside in. When all the roots had broken, they pushed the island down the lake to an uninhabited bay.

That year, Herb had shot a bear the previous winter and promised Dad to serve bear meat for dinner the last night we were in camp. He took the *Daisy Mae* in to Fort Francis to get supplies and bring the bear meat from the storage freezer. He did not make it back to camp before we left. Dad learned later that Herb and the Indian man he took with him had gotten drunk and the Indian had done a war dance on top of someone's car so they were both in jail sobering up when we went through Fort Francis on the way home.

Coach Sarr had quit going to Camp Manitou and was spending his summers fishing in Canada. He told Dad about Lake of the Woods, about fifty miles northwest of the Rainy Lake region. Dad decided to take Bruce and me to Coach Sarr's favorite place at Sioux Narrows on Lake of the Woods rather than return to Pioneer Lodge. Sioux Narrows was on the road and therefore more accessible. The lodge there had electricity, plumbing, better boats, and good guides, so we had a good time fishing there.

Dad taught us how to use tools and make things. The Optimist Club in Normal started a soapbox derby. Bruce found out about it and wanted to enter. Dad showed him how to saw one-by-four boards and nail them to cross boards to make the floor of a racer. He taught Bruce how to clamp axle rods to 1 X 4s to hold the wheels. One of these axle boards was nailed to the back of the floor. The other was mounted to the front end of the floor with a single bolt and washers so it could turn and steer the car using ropes attached to the axle boards.

There was a gap in one plank in the center of the floor. A board was attached to the front end of the hole with a hinge. A rubber shoe heel was nailed to the bottom of the other end of the board. A spring was rigged to hold the board off the ground. This board was the brake for the car. Bruce built a box for the front end body and a smaller box for the rear end body.

We were limited in Normal to ten-inch wheels. (The soapbox derby in Akron, Ohio, uses fourteen-inch roller bearing wheels.) Dad took Bruce to the local junk dealer and bought four used wheels with brass bushings and hard rubber tires. Bruce and I spent hours in the basement polishing the axle bars so the wheels would spin more freely. We would polish the axle with emery paper, apply copious graphite oil, and then spin the tires and time them until they stopped. We kept polishing the axles until the spin time would not increase.

Dad followed this construction closely and gave us instructions for improvements. I worked with Bruce for the entire project. Several other boys in the neighborhood built cars and wanted to try them out before the race.

There was a hill that was a block long on a little used straight street about two blocks from our house. With a driver steering, we pushed the racers over to the hill and started them with a single push to see how far they would go past the bottom of the hill. Some cars went farther than others, but we could not standardize the push start so we did not know which racer was fastest.

The official race was held on that same hill, but the Optimists had built a starting ramp that started two racers simultaneously. The cars were timed to the finish line. Bruce came in somewhere in the middle of the group. The boy who won had a plank with a fixed rear axle and a moveable front axle, which he steered by lying on the plank and holding the axle in his hands. He braked by dragging the toes of his tennis shoes. The next year, the rules were much more detailed about racer design, steering, and brakes.

Several of the racers had official ten-inch soapbox derby ball bearing wheels from Akron, Ohio. They had a definite advantage. Dad wanted to encourage Bruce, so the next year, he bought him some ball bearing wheels. He bought them from the same junk dealer; the junk man convinced Bruce that the new tires were too wide so they would drag on the racer. He said that they needed to be trimmed down to reduce the drag. The dealer could have that done for Bruce, so Bruce had him do it. The dealer procrastinated too long, and Bruce did not get the wheels until the day before the racers were impounded for inspection before the race. He put the wheels on the racer, but he did not get a chance to try the new wheels.

I inherited Bruce's old wheels and build a racer for myself. I used the same basic design, but tapered the front of the racer from the middle of the front to both sides. Instead of a box for the body, I made an arch that I attached to the floor in front of the seat. I ran heavy twine from the edge of the floor to the arch. I wrapped old drapery fabric over the strings to make the body. I mounted a vertical board behind the seat and stretched the drapery fabric from the board to the flooring in back. At Dad's suggestion, I spray painted the whole car blue except the wheels and axles. I used the spray-painting attachment for my mother's vacuum cleaner. She was not too happy about that when she found out. I cut out letters and pinned them to the fabric as stencils to spell John's Jalopy on the fabric when they were removed.

The Optimists had built a much higher ramp with a better release mechanism. Bruce was one of the first racers to run. His racer came off the ramp and immediately started to slow down. He did not make it to the bottom the hill and the finish line. His narrowed tires had collapsed and gone flat. This made it hard to steer, and steering straight was crucial in this race to maintain speed. Each car ran twice, so the second time, Bruce was ready for the steering problem and made it to the finish line, but just barely.

Using Bruce's cast off wheels, and learning about the steering problem before I went down, I came in fourth of about twenty-five racers. Bruce was so upset over the way he had been sold on narrowing the tires that he did not come to the awards ceremony. Dad was so mad at the junk dealer for ruining the tires that he never did business with him again.

The next summer, I did not enter the race. Dr. Rose Parker had other plans for me. She was professor of education and psychology at Illinois State Normal University in Normal. She and her mother and sister often looked after Bruce and me when our parents were out of town. She convinced Mom and Dad that I was under the shadow of Bruce and needed to have time away from him. She also wanted a companion on a trip to visit her sister in New Mexico.

Rose did not want to travel alone and had been having some health problems. She had a new Hudson sedan with a semiautomatic transmission that did not work well and might leave her stranded. She was also afraid that she would have a medical problem and could not get to help, so she taught me how to drive her car as we went across the desert. She would have me sit on a cushion behind the wheel and steer while she had her foot on the gas. Eventually, she let me handle the gas pedal and steer. Rose convinced me that Dad should never know that I had my first driving lesson when I was ten.

I was officially the cat sitter. Rose had an eighteen-year-old Persian cat that she took with her. My job was to set out the pan with kitty litter in the motel every night and empty it in the morning. I spent a month with Rose and her sister Dolores and Dolores's husband Joel. He was a rocket scientist at White Sands Proving Grounds near Las Curses, New Mexico. He was in charge of monitoring two missile launches each year from a trailer full of electronics.

Rose wanted to buy me cowboy boots, but Dad thought they would damage my feet. He said it would be all right for me to get good riding boots. They did not have that type of boots in Juarez, so I wound up with cowboy boots after all. Dad was not happy when I returned home with cowboy boots.

I had a great time visiting Juarez, Mexico, and exploring the New Mexico desert. I do not know what it did for the problem Rose thought I had.

Chapter 15

My father was very committed to his patients and made house calls until he retired. He charged $8 for many years, but increased to $10 about two years before he retired. Office visits were $5.

He would often be called into the country to see someone who was too sick to come to the office. He cared for many of the local farmers and their families. Dad never had difficulty finding a farm on which to hunt pheasants in the fall. He took Bruce and me with him after we were twelve years old. He taught us how to hunt pheasants and quail in the cornfields and forests.

Noon on November 11 was the opening day of pheasant season every year. Dad always took us to the Gertsons' farm for the first day. He had cared for both Mr. and Mrs. Gertson for many years, and they insisted that he hunt at their farm on opening day. Mrs. Gertson would prepare an early lunch so we could start hunting at noon. The lunch always had chicken, ham, and beef with lots of potatoes and gravy and several vegetables. This was followed by cake and pie. After that huge lunch, we felt more like taking a nap than hunting.

The first year I went with Dad, we saw a fox running across a plowed field next to the stubble field we were hunting. Mr. Gertson hated foxes because they killed his chickens. He told us to shoot the fox. Bruce and I each emptied our shotguns (three shots each) at the fox. We could see the shot pattern in the plowed ground surrounding the fox and we hit it with each shot, but Bruce had to reload with a seventh shell to finally kill the fox. Dad remarked that we were both good shots, but it took a lot of birdshot to kill a fox. Mr. Gertson hung the fox on a fence to show the neighborhood that one fox was dead.

Every fall, before hunting season, Dad would buy several boxes of shotgun shells and two big boxes of clay pigeons. He had his own spring-loaded trap to throw the pigeons. We would go to the farm of one of his patients in the Mackinaw river bottoms. We would spread a blanket on the ground in a stubble field or picked cornfield for everyone to lay their guns on so only the shooter held a gun. The trap would be set off to the side where the shooter could not see it throw the discs. We would take turns shooting several clay pigeons each or working the trap.

As soon as the first shot was fired, pickup trucks would start appearing over the surrounding hills. The local farmers came to "watch," but as soon as Dad asked them if they wanted to shoot a few, a shotgun would materialize from under the seat of their pickup truck.

Dad furnished the shells and clay pigeons. Bruce had both .410-gauge and .16-gauge shotguns; I had a .16-gauge, identical to Bruce's; and Dad had several .12-gauge shotguns, so we had a wide variety of shells available. By the time we rotated through the assembled shooters, there were not many turns for Dad, Bruce, or me, but everyone had a good time. After a few years, someone determined that the remnants of the clay pigeons were toxic to pigs. Most of the farmers ran pigs in their cornfields after the corn was picked, so the shooting was somewhat curtailed.

Dad had a Model 12 pump shotgun that he preferred. He told us that he had owned a Model 12 Winchester shotgun in the 1930s that had a serial number less than 800. He had traded it to Shorty Peyton, the local barbershop owner, for another shotgun. He regretted the trade when he found out that Model 12s with serial numbers under 1000 were very valuable. He owned a number of shotguns, trying to find a semiautomatic shotgun that handled like a Model 12 pump.

Dad liked to hunt quail. To do it right, he decided he needed a bird dog. His friend Les Cornick had furnished room and board for a college student at ISNU named Darrel Ebkin, in exchange for work in his appliance business. Darrel was now a hog farmer in southern Illinois and knew people who raised, trained, and sold hunting dogs. Dad and Les went to visit Darrel at his farm, and Darrel connected them with his favorite hunting dog breeder. Dad chose a puppy that had not been trained and arranged to pick him up after he was trained.

When Dad went back in the fall to pick up the dog, the breeder took him out to the fields to watch the dog work. The breeder told Dad to work the dog while he sat in his pickup truck. The trainer could not walk with the dogs because he had a painful ingrown toenail. He explained that he was too busy to have it cut out and was just limping along until the time was right.

Dad asked him if he had any alcohol in his truck. The trainer pulled out a partial fifth of Jim Beam from under the seat of his truck and said that was the only thing he had. Dad insisted that it would work fine. He told the trainer to drink some before he splashed some on the blade of his pocketknife and some on the big toe and proceeded to cut out the ingrown toenail. Dad always carried a pocketknife and kept the blade super sharp. He was from an age of surgeons who prided themselves in being able to perform any surgery with the tools available.

Zip, the bird dog, worked very well the first season when Dad took him hunting. After hunting season, Dad kept Zip in the house and treated him like a house dog. After that, Zip lost his ability to point and hold birds. Many people told Dad that keeping a bird dog as a house dog would ruin the dog for hunting, but he would never keep Zip outdoors in a kennel, especially during the winter. Dad treated Zip as a house dog.

When they moved to Arkansas, Zip had the run of the neighborhood. One day, he came home with a live duck in his mouth. Zip would put the duck down and follow it around the yard. Every few minutes, he would pick up the duck and carry it to another part of the yard. Dad saw him and took the duck away. He knew where the farmer lived who kept ducks about a quarter of a mile away, so he took the duck back. Zip did this several times, but never hurt any of the ducks. He just played with them.

One day, some animal got into the duck cage and killed several of the ducks. The farmer went to the local constable and demanded that Zip be put to sleep for killing his ducks. Since Zip had never hurt one of the ducks, Dad fought the idea, but the farmer was insistent even though he had not seen Zip kill a duck. Dad was sure that a fox or raccoon had killed the ducks, but could not convince the farmer. The constable sided with the farmer against the newcomer snowbird, but agreed not to have Zip killed if Dad would give Zip away to someone who lived more than ten miles away. Dad found Zip a home, but it really upset him to lose his dog.

Chapter 16

Dad told stories of going out into the country at night to see patients. He often had trouble finding the right farmhouse so he learned to have them turn on the porch light or the pole light at the barn or tie a rag on the mailbox. He would examine the patient in bed or on the kitchen table to decide if they needed medical treatment like oral medication or a shot of penicillin or if they needed to be in the hospital. He always kept a pillow and a blanket in the backseat of his car so he could bring patients to the hospital. He usually drove a four-door car so that patients could get in and out of the backseat.

I remember one night when he had to drive out into the country in a dense fog. He could barely see the road to keep out of the ditch. Fortunately, most of the country roads in central Illinois are very straight. Suddenly, there was a huge hog in the road in front of his car. It was too close for him to stop before hitting the sow and rolling it down the road. He got out of the car and checked the hog and determined that it was dead. He looked around for the nearest farmhouse to find the owner of the hog.

When he told the farmer that he had killed the sow, the farmer got mad and wanted my dad to pay for the "championship" hog that was going to win prizes at the state fair. My father replied that if the hog was so valuable, he should have taken better care of it and not let it run in the road in the fog. I think my dad gave him the price of an average hog and told him to repair his fences with the money.

When he made these house calls in the country at night for a bellyache, he would have to make the decision after examining the patient whether they had a "surgical belly" or "nonsurgical belly." If he thought they had a surgical abdomen, he would load the patient into his car and drive to the nearest house with a telephone to call the hospital to alert them that he needed the surgical team. Then he would drive the patient to the hospital. The nurses would meet him at the emergency entrance with a gurney for the patient. The nurses and the anesthesiologist would prepare the patient for surgery while he changed into scrubs.

In the absence of sophisticated X-rays, CT scans, and MRIs he would have to decide if the patient had indigestion, stomach flu, or a kidney stone that were medical, or a bowel obstruction, appendicitis, gallbladder attack, or infarcted intestine that were causes for surgery. These latter diagnoses fall into the category of an acute abdomen. The treatment in those days was to open up the abdomen and explore to find out what was wrong. Appendicitis had several distinct physical findings that told the surgeon to make his incision at McBurney's point rather than the exploratory incision in the midline of the abdomen. He had to rely on his abilities of physical examination and diagnosis.

One of the cases that haunted Dad was that of a good friend. The woman was pregnant with her third child. She went into labor two months before term and delivered a girl who was very premature. The infant developed hyaline membrane disease of prematurity. This is a disease of the lungs that prevents the child from getting oxygen. The treatment of that disease is to give the child 100 percent oxygen using a ventilator.

If a premature baby receives too much oxygen at the exact time when the membranes spontaneously dissolve, they may alter the development of the retina in the eye. Fibrous bands develop where the retinal vessels are still growing to supply oxygen to the retina. These bands shrink with time, pulling the retina into a mass in the center of the eye, resulting in blindness.

At the time this baby was born, the causal relationship between oxygen and the subsequent blindness had not been established. The first publication connecting oxygen to the blindness called retinitis of prematurity came out of Australia about a year after she was born, about the time her blindness was complete.

When my father found out that his treatment to save Sue's life had caused the blindness, he told the parents. They were happy that Sue had survived and did not blame Dad because the blindness was a complication of the life-saving oxygen therapy. He felt guilty and made sure that the child received the best medical care.

Her parents placed her in a school for the blind where she learned mobility, self-confidence, and Braille. Her father was a ham radio operator. She rapidly learned code and was an accomplished radio ham by the time she was twelve years old. She invited Dad to her high school graduation. She eventually obtained a college education and married a salmon fisherman in Alaska. Her parents told me that she would often go fishing with her husband and helped with the fish and the boat. It is hard to comprehend how a blind person could work on a boat that is unsteady and often quite dangerous, even for sighted people. I found a letter from her to my dad congratulating him when he passed his novice ham radio license exam after he retired.

Shortly before Dad retired, he saw the wife of the former sheriff of McLean County in his office. After he examined her and prescribed her mediations, she opened her purse and pulled out a pistol and a bag of bullets. She handed them to Dad and told him that Sheriff

Rader had told her before he died that he wanted Dad to have his service revolver.

In about 1938, thieves had stolen a car in Normal and were headed north out of town. The sheriff intercepted them at the Little Red School House on the extension of Linden Street, about a mile north of Normal. The "shootout at the Little Red Schoolhouse" resulted in the capturing of the wounded thieves. Sheriff Rader had received three gunshot wounds to his limbs. Dad removed the bullets from the sheriff after the gun battle, and he survived for many years.

One day when we were driving around Normal after he retired, he told me about a man who lived on Broadway a few blocks from our house. The man had called him at two o'clock in the morning complaining that he was doubled up with abdominal pain. Dad rolled out and went to see him. He had a hard, tender abdomen, so Dad took him to the hospital and opened him up. He found a mesenteric infarction involving the blood supply to six feet of his small intestine, causing death of the intestine. He resected the six feet of bowel, reconnecting the remaining ends. The man lived for several years afterward.

On that same drive, Dad pointed out a house where a woman lived who, he said, had the largest uterine fibroids that he had ever removed. This reminded me of the time, years before, when he was reading the current issue of *The Journal of Obstetrics and Gynecology* that he always kept in the stack of journals next to his recliner. He was reading an article about removal of a large ovarian tumor when he complained that the professors were always looking for something to publish. He had removed an ovarian tumor twice that size a few months before.

Dad was eating lunch one day when the phone rang. It was from the hospital. An ambulance had been sent to a farm near Mclean,

Illinois, about thirty miles away. A young man had driven his motorcycle to the farmhouse to pick up his girlfriend to take her for a ride. When he came back out the lane about fifteen minutes later, with his girlfriend riding behind him on his motorcycle, someone had stretched a barbed wire across the gate to keep the cows in. He did not see the wire, so they hit the wire going about twenty-five miles per hour. The wire caught them both just below the chin and had cut both of them very deeply. The ambulance was bringing them to Brokaw Hospital.

Dad hung up and called our neighbor, Dr. Earl Hartenbauer, the only eye, ear, nose, and throat doctor in town who lived two doors down the street. They agreed to meet immediately at the hospital. Dad then went to his study and pulled his copy of *Grey's Anatomy* from the shelf and left for the hospital.

The two doctors, working in operating rooms that were side by side, operated all afternoon sewing up the two patients. They went back and forth, helping each other. He told me that the wire had cut through the trachea (windpipe) and esophagus, but had been stopped by the front of the spine. The wire had not cut any of the major arteries or veins on either patient, so blood loss was not severe. Most of the muscles of the front half of the neck had been severed. The doctors used the anatomy book to identify the two ends of the many cut strap muscles of the neck to reattach the correct cut ends.

The recurrent laryngeal nerves that control the vocal cords branch from the Vegas nerve in the neck. They loop below the aorta and the subclavian arteries near the heart and ascend along the trachea to the vocal cords in the larynx (voice box). These had been cut with the trachea, so neither patient would be able to talk naturally again. Both patients survived.

Years later, I was in Cohen's Drugstore in Normal with my dad. A man recognized my dad and approached him. He held up a thing that looked like an old electric shaver to the side of his neck and said, "Doc, you probably do not remember me, but I am the guy who ran into the wire years ago, near McLean. You had to sew me and my girlfriend back together. I am forever grateful for what you did for me that afternoon." My dad did not recognize him after all the years, but remembered the situation and was pleased to be recognized and thanked. The man was using a buzzer that was invented by Bell Laboratories. When held against his larynx, it vibrated the voice box and vocal cords so that he could talk. It sounded like an early computer-generated monotone voice.

In the late forties, Dad brought home some long wire loops from the office. These were made of quarter-inch steel rod and were from three to five feet long and eight to ten inches wide. One end was bent in to form an M shape. The other end was wider and curved in slightly and was padded with gauze wrapped around it as padding. I asked Dad what these were for, so he explained that they were for setting broken bones.

When a patient had a broken hip or shoulder, the muscles on the leg and hip, or arm, would go into spasm, pulling the ends of the bone together, causing the broken bone ends to overlap. The fracture could not be reduced and set until the muscles relaxed.

Dad had a metal shop make these loops for him. The padded end of this loop was placed in the groin, or armpit, with the loop extending past the foot or elbow. The foot and ankle, or arm, were wrapped with gauze that made a loop around the inward curve of the other end of the loop. A stick was placed through this gauze loop and twisted to tighten the loop and pull on the leg. As the muscles relaxed, the loop was twisted more to tighten the pull. When the muscles had relaxed enough, the arm or leg could be manipulated to set the fracture. The limb could be held in position by the loop of metal or a cast was applied, depending on the location of the fracture.

Dad explained that an orthopedic surgeon had moved to Normal, so he would not be setting this type of fracture anymore. He wanted to keep these loops in the attic until he was sure that the orthopedist would stay in Normal.

Chapter 17

Dad's office was in the middle of downtown Normal. It was upstairs above the Normal Public Library. Across the hall was the office of Dr. Ray Dowd, who was about the same age as my father. They often covered for each other if one was out of town or had a serious commitment. There were at least twenty steps because of the high ceiling of the public library below. The building did not have an elevator, so house calls were made on patients who could not climb the steps.

The door was on the right at the top of the steps. After entering, there was a long hallway that led back toward the street into a large waiting room lined with an assortment of chairs. There were stacks of old magazines from home on a central table. Dad always kept a large book in the waiting room. It was about an inch thick and contained the latest cartoons from *The New Yorker* magazine. This waiting room and a treatment room faced North Street.

From the waiting room, a door led away from the street to a triangular room with a big desk and file cabinets—the business office. Two doors off this room led to exam rooms. Between the two exam rooms was a laboratory room with a counter holding a microscope and an ashtray. There was another counter with a sink and a centrifuge. A telephone hung on the wall above the ashtray. Dad could take calls in the laboratory with some privacy.

Dad smoked, so as he would go back and forth between patients in the exam rooms, through the lab, he would look in the microscope where his nurse often put a slide with urine sediment or a blood smear for him to examine and record his findings. He would often light a cigarette and take a few drags. He would put the cigarette in the ashtray and go to the next patient. When he came back through, he would take a few drags in passing before seeing the next patient. He would get four to six drags from each cigarette before it burned out. We calculated that he went through one and a half packs per afternoon but actually smoked less than one pack per afternoon. He was slow to switch to filter cigarettes when they became available. I think Camel cigarettes, his favorite, were about the last to add filters. So many of his patients smoked cigarettes in those days that most of them did not notice the smoke on his breath.

Dad had a diathermy machine in the treatment room that he used for treatment of chronic back pain. People would lie on their stomach on a treatment table with a panel from the machine on their back. The patients swore that a half hour under the machine relieved their back pain. Usually his nurse handled the diathermy treatments without Dad even seeing them. Patients would drop in to request a treatment, so she would put them in that room and set up the therapy.

There was a silver sterilizer in one treatment room that had boiling water in it when the office was in operation. The tray in the boiling water lifted out when the lid was opened. Syringes, needles, and various surgical instruments were kept in the boiling water for sterilization. Instruments were removed using sterile tongs and placed on sterile towels to dry and cool.

A white porcelain treatment table in each room had three large clear bottles across the back. One had purple gentian violet; the second had orange potassium permanganate solution; the third bottle contained clear or light blue denatured alcohol. He used these solutions to clean and sterilize the skin area around cuts and abrasions. He often put stitches in lacerations in his office.

He had a treatment that I heard about from his patients, but never saw him perform. This involved rods about eight inches long that were curved on one end. He would wrap gauze or cotton around the curved end of the rod and then pour permanganate solution into a tray. The cotton tips would be dipped in the permanganate solution and then swabbed on the back of the throat and the back side of the soft palate. Patients would choke and gag and vow that they would never come back.

The high school principal described this procedure to me as "barbaric." This was a miracle cure for a bad cold with a postnasal drip. The next day, these same patients would be singing his praise and recommending the treatment to all of their friends.

When Bruce or I felt sick in school, we would go to Dad's office on the way home. He would see us at the end of his schedule and take us home. We went to the office rather than wait for Dad to come home because Cleta Little, his longtime office nurse, was better at giving shots than Dad was. She always made sure that the needle was sharp and had more gentle touch at giving injections.

In those days, needles were sterilized and reused and sometimes were resharpened when they became dull. Dad always wiped the needle through a sterile cotton ball to see if there was a barb on the needle that would pull out strands of cotton.

If the needle hit a hard surface, the tip would curl back and create a barb that made the needle dull and hurt when it was pulled out. He kept the needles in special test tubes with a constricted neck that held the tip of the needle from hitting the end of the test tube, dulling it. The tubes were plugged with a cotton ball to keep the needle in the tube but allow steam to enter the tube during sterilization. In my memory, we got a lot of penicillin shots! I think that most of the illnesses were viral, but on the other hand, we never got rheumatic fever from an undertreated strep throat.

One of Bruce's best friends had rheumatic fever from a strep infection. He developed heart problems from rheumatic fever, secondary to a strep throat. He was so weak that he missed school for a year. He recovered and went on to become the president of State Farm Insurance.

Dad had to put stitches in me several times. During the summer, after I was in the seventh grade, I hung out at the country club, swimming, golfing, and occasionally caddying. One day I was sitting in the caddie shack, hoping to make some money carrying clubs. The caddie master called me to shag golf balls on the driving range for a member.

It was a hot, sunny day so I stood under a big maple tree. The man would hit balls that landed short of the tree and rolled into the shade under the tree where I picked them up. I saw him change clubs, but he did not indicate whether he had a longer or shorter club. He hit the first ball that went high and disappeared behind the leaves of the tree. The next thing I knew, it crashed through the tree right above me and hit me square in the nose, right between the eyes. I felt pain and bent over with my hands in front of my face. My hands were quickly covered with blood. I ran for the pro shop and told the caddie master to call my dad.

The man who hit the ball came into the shop at that time and told me that I should not try to catch the balls. When the caddie master asked for my dad's number, the golfer yelled, "Don't call his dad, call a doctor!" The golfer did not know who my father was. The caddie master put ice in a towel for me to hold on my nose to get the bleeding stopped. My dad was in surgery, so he called my mom who came to get me and take me to the hospital. They took X-rays of my nose, and I waited for my dad to come in to stitch my nose.

Dad arrived in about two hours and stitched the laceration on the bridge of my nose. The radiologist said that the bridge of my nose was fractured, but not displaced. Dad packed my nose to stabilize the fracture and sent me home. Dr. Hartenbauer dropped in after work and looked in my nose and said everything would be all right without any surgery.

The other time Dad had to stitch me up was when I was in eighth grade. I was acting in a play that was to be presented at the high school, which was about six blocks from the grade school. Everyone in the play walked to the high school at about 10:00 a.m. for a rehearsal on the stage. It was a snowy morning with ice on the sidewalks. Kids were throwing snowballs. I ducked a snowball and slipped on the ice. There was a low pipe railing along the sidewalk to keep people off the grass. It had a metal strip on top of the pipe with little iron pyramids about every two inches to keep people from sitting on the railing while they waited for a bus. My right knee landed on one of those pyramids, and it really hurt. I was still able to walk, so I kept walking to the high school.

By the time I got to the stage, I was limping a little. One of my friends asked me what happened, so I told him. He wanted to see my knee, so I pulled up my pants. I saw blood running down my shin, so I showed it to my teacher.

The stage of the auditorium was also the basketball floor of the combined auditorium/gymnasium. The locker rooms and training room for basketball were right next to the auditorium. They took me to the training room where the coach looked at my knee. I had split the skin over my kneecap all the way to the kneecap itself. It was a three-corner tear about two inches long.

My mother was on the school board and my brother was in high school, so they knew who my father was and called his office. Again, he was in surgery. My mother drove to the high school and took me to Dad's office where we waited about two hours for my father to sew me up. Patients came before family.

When I was a freshman in high school, Dad let me go out for football. I was a little heavy and out of shape, but I played center on the freshman team. Dad did not want me to become flat footed, so I had to wear arch supports in my football shoes. My helmet was made of leather and was so old and soft that I could fold the earflaps into the crown and fold the crown almost flat to put it on the shelf in my locker. The varsity had new hard plastic helmets, but freshmen used the old ones.

My knees got banged up a lot playing center and guard. At the end of football season, my left knee swelled to about twice the normal size and hurt when I climbed stairs.

Dad took me down to the office on Saturday morning and examined the knee. He thought it was full of fluid and decided to drain it. Cleta was there to assist. He injected some Novocain at the point where he would put the drainage needle. He had me sit up so I could watch him. Cleta prepped the area with permanganate. Dad put the largest hypodermic needle that I had ever seen on a large syringe. He shoved the needle through the numbed area of skin and pushed it into the knee joint. It was painless, but felt strange, like pressure. He proceeded to draw about two ounces of straw-colored fluid from my knee, squirting it into a narrow graduated glass cylinder to measure the volume.

Dad put a Band-Aid over the puncture site and told me to stand up. Once I was standing, Cleta looked at me and told me to sit down immediately and put my head down between my knees. I felt woozy and started seeing spots, so I sat down before I passed out. She told me that I was white as a sheet. After about five minutes with my head between my knees, they had me sit up. Everything felt all right then, so I stood up and did not feel faint. I think Dad wanted me to watch him so I would develop an interest in medicine. The fainting spell had the opposite effect.

My knee continued to bother me, and I developed tender bumps below both kneecaps. Dad took me to see one of his classmates from medical school, Dr. H. R. McCarroll. He was an orthopedist in St. Louis. He had me get X-rays of both knees and concluded that I had two small extra bones in my left knee, behind the patella (kneecap).

I also had Osgood-Schlatter disease, which consists of inflammation that causes tenderness and pain at the tibial tuberosity, the bump, about three inches below the knee, where the patellar tendon inserts into the tibia (shin bone). This is a disease that is not unusual in boys during puberty and goes away with time.

Dad decided that participation in sports would be bad for my knees. He pulled me out of all physical education for the rest of high school for medical reasons. I still played in the band and walked a mile each way to and from school, weather permitting, so I got plenty of exercise. I spent the physical education period each day as a messenger for the principal's office.

Dad and Dr. Doud, who had the office across the hall from Dad's, had a problem finding a parking place near the office. Normal had free parking and was a busy little community. There was a drugstore and a beauty shop on the corner next to the offices. They appealed to the city council and had two parking places at the corner designated for doctors only. Some people did not pay attention to the signs, so Dad had to often park somewhere else.

The post office for Normal was located directly across the street from Dad's office. There was a drive-up drop box in front of the post office so about half of a block was marked No Parking. If the two doctor parking spaces were full, Dad would drive in front of the post office and pull forward past the drop box so that cars had access to the box. He would leave his car there all afternoon. He had a metal shield with a caduceus and the letters MD attached to his license plate, but he would occasionally get a ticket for illegal parking. The wife of the police chief was the bookkeeper for his practice, so he would give the ticket to her and never had a problem.

Living in a farm community, we often received gifts of fresh sweet corn and vegetables from some patient's garden. Patients would bring them to the office or leave them at our front door. Dad would get a call from a patient asking if we would be home: they had just butchered and wanted to drop off some steaks or chops for us, but the meat needed to go into the freezer right away so they wanted to be sure that we were at home when it was delivered.

Dad was very flexible about how he was paid. I do not know if it was Mom or Dad who arranged this, but at the end of eighth grade, Mom told me that I could quit piano lessons if I took up marimba. I was already playing the drums, and the marimba is one of the percussion instruments. I was getting nowhere learning to play the piano (seven years of lessons and only in the third-year book), so I agreed to the switch. Dad told me that he had a patient who had an old marimba that he no longer played. He wanted Dad to take the marimba in payment for his recent surgery. Dad agreed to take the marimba, so we went to pick it up.

This marimba had dull nickel plated resonators and a natural wooden rack for wooden keys, probably make of oak. The frame was nickel plated tubing and metal straps with big rubber-treaded wheels. It was perfectly good for a beginner and had a nice tone. I think it was a setup for me, but I liked the marimba much better than the piano. Bruce did not play the marimba, so this differentiated us as percussionists.

Dad practiced in a small- to medium-sized community and had great empathy for his patients. He practiced before Medicare and Medicaid. He had many elderly patients who were on social security or a pension that furnished a limited fixed income. Although his fees were modest, he had many patients who told him that they could not afford to pay him for surgery, after the surgery, and after they had received his bill. He knew which patients were really unable to pay. He would tell those patients that they should "pay what you can and I will charge the rest of the bill to the dust to let the rain settle it."

Mom ran the billing process and hand typed the bills. Bruce and I would stuff bills into envelopes, seal the envelopes and put stamps on them. If there was a bill that was several months past due, Mom would watch the newspapers. The *Normalite*, which came out once a week, was full of gossip. The *Bloomington Daily Pantograph* often ran small articles about business transactions and unusual vacations. Mom would clip articles about vacations and large expenditures by Dad's patients. If they had an outstanding balance, she would staple the article to the bill. People who had just returned from two weeks in Miami usually paid up quickly when they received this reminder. The town was too small for anyone to hide.

Dad had certain patients whom he knew could not pay, but he cared for them and wrote off the fees. This influenced me in my practice. I ran indigent clinics throughout my career at both the

University of Texas in Galveston and St. Francis Medical Center in Pittsburgh. The care was usually covered by hospital or state funds for these patients. I was paid a salary for this care. With my private patients, I never balance billed above the amounts that Medicare or private insurance allowed. The law requires that doctors collect the 20 percent that Medicare allows but does not pay. Some doctors try to collect the difference between their fee and the allowable amount. I knew that my father and thousands of prior practitioners would roll over in their graves if I tried to do that.

Chapter 18

Dad was very proud of his oldest son who was majoring in premed studies and planned to become a doctor. He hoped Bruce would eventually come home and take over his practice. Bruce had tied for the highest grades in the high school his senior year, and Dad was sure that he would do well in college.

I was doing well in school and liked math and science. I thought I wanted to be a project coordinator in the space program. Space exploration had just begun and had a bright future. With one son on the way to becoming a doctor, Dad did not push me in any way to go into medicine. Dad actually seemed to be in favor of my becoming an engineer.

Dad's medical practice was very busy and had priority over everything else. Mom was in charge of getting us places and making sure that we got things done on time. Dad tried to make it to band performances and plays, but always came in his own car in case he had an emergency. This was before the age of beepers and cell phones, so he left telephone numbers where he could be reached. He was paged at football and basketball games and got aisle seats in theaters so the ushers could find him. He probably missed as many high school events as he made because of patient needs.

I remember sitting next to him in the auditorium for high school graduation when I was in eighth grade. My mother was on Dad's other side, and Bruce was in the band. As they announced the name of the graduate, Dad would turn to my mother and say something like, "I delivered her" or "I set his fractured arm last summer when he fell off a horse."

My mother would reply with something like, "Yes, and they haven't paid for it yet." It was a small town, and many of the graduates were his patients.

This familiarity with his patients and the ubiquity of his patients in this small town was good and bad. There was a girl in high school who used to tease me by saying "I know something about you. Your dad told us something about you."

I found out that she was in the exam room when my dad saw her little brother. My dad had obviously tried to reassure her mother by telling her that I had, or had done, something like her son. My dad knew so little about who were my classmates that I don't think he ever considered it getting back to me. I never did find out what it was that she was teasing me about.

Dad was one of three general practitioners in Normal and my mother was on the local school board, so Bruce and I were well known in town. We could not get away with anything. If we climbed a fence or picked some cherries from a neighbor's tree, Mom knew about it before we got home. As soon as Dad got home, he knew about it, but he left discipline to Mom unless it was really serious.

We ate dinner at home almost every night, and it was a family affair. Bruce and I were quizzed about school—what we were doing in class and after school activities, what happened at school like the announcements in home room, gossip, and who our friends were. Both Mom and Dad commented freely about these. We knew how they felt about everything and were often told how to handle situations. Both parents had strong opinions of the morality and the appropriateness of actions and responses.

Dad would tell Mom about his patients, and Mom would tell him what was happening on the school board, the church, and various clubs. As far as Bruce and I were concerned, the family kept very few secrets internally, but anything said about patients was not to be repeated.

Dad was very sensitive about being one of the wealthiest people in town. We had a very nice house and belonged to Bloomington Country Club. Dad always drove either a Chevrolet sedan or a bottom-of-the-line Buick special. Mom drove a 1940 Chevy coupe until 1951 when she got a Chevrolet station wagon so she could haul Bruce's drum set. She graduated to an Oldsmobile 88 Holiday coupe in 1955 and gave the station wagon to Bruce for college. A year later, when my new marimba would not fit in the trunk of the '88, we took the carrying cases to the dealer to see what would hold the marimba. She bought a '98 Oldsmobile sedan to get a trunk large enough to carry the knocked-down marimba.

Bruce and I wore gabardine pants and cotton shirts with collars to school. Mom would not let us wear jeans or T-shirts to school. We always went to Marben's clothing, a block off the courthouse square in Bloomington. They specialized in work clothes and inexpensive casual clothes. We got sport coats to wear to church from a better clothing store where Dad bought his suits.

Dad would wear his suits for years until they got shiny. He would not get a new hat until he wore out the crown where he held it when he put it on and took it off. He did like Italian Borsalino hats that he had cleaned and blocked once a year at the hat shop on Main Street in Bloomington. Mom would nag him to get new clothes, but Dad told her he would wear them until they had holes. He did not need to be a fashion plate.

When Bruce and I were in high school, Dad told us not to look for summer jobs. He thought that there were too many people our age who needed jobs to make money for college. We were not allowed to compete with them because Dad assured us that he would pay for our college education.

The exception to ostentation was when Bruce wanted and got an English bicycle for his twelfth birthday. Three years later, I got my English bicycle for my twelfth birthday. They were the only English bicycles in Normal. We caught a lot of grief over our skinny-wheeled bicycles. Everyone else wanted a big Schwinn Roadster bike.

Mom had a nonmedical remedy for her migraine headaches. She would go to one of the department stores in downtown Bloomington to buy a new dress or hat. She said that it made her feel better. One weekend, she and Dad went to Chicago and came home with a cinnamon-colored mink stole. She was the talk of the church for at least a week.

When I was in high school, Mom went to Chicago and bought a Black Mercedes sedan with red leather interior. Dad did not object, but he continued to drive his modest cars. The Mercedes had a shift stick on the steering column, but no clutch on the floor. Whenever the shift stick was moved, the clutch automatically engaged for the shift. Unfortunately, this shift mechanism did not work very well, so I had to drive the Mercedes to Oak Park, outside Chicago, twice for repairs—all the way in second gear. Staying in second gear made acceleration from stoplights difficult and high speeds on US 66 impossible. She eventually traded it for an Oldsmobile.

When Bruce graduated from high school, he was planning to major in premed at the University of Colorado. My parents did not realize that the University of Colorado was voted the biggest party school in the country at that time. When we went to Boulder, Colorado, that summer to see the university, Dad insisted on stopping at the University of Colorado Medical School in Denver.

It was midsummer, so the medical school building was nearly deserted. We walked around in the school, looking into laboratories and classrooms. We came to some double doors marked "Anatomy Laboratory: Positively No Admission without Permission of Denver County Sheriff."

Dad said, "Good, here is the anatomy lab. Let's see what they are doing."

He barged right in and told us to follow him. I was sure that we were going to land in jail, but we followed him. There was no one in the lab, so Dad walked up to one of the tables and zipped open the body bag. The body in the bag was partially dissected, so he started to point out body parts to Bruce. I hung back and kept watching the door. After a few minutes, Dad zipped up the bag and we left.

When I expressed my worries to dad, he told me that because he was a doctor, he was allowed to go into anatomy labs. I guess Bruce passed his "doctor test" by not passing out or throwing up when Dad opened the body bag.

When Bruce was at the university, he wrote frequent letters home. He talked about his experiences in the Colorado marching band, playing tennis after shoveling snow from the court, and fraternity activities, but very little about his classes. When his grades came in the mail to my parents, they remarked that he was doing very well. After his second semester, my dad commented that there were no science courses on the list of grades. Bruce was home then and explained to Dad that the university wanted doctors to be well-educated citizens, so they incorporated lots of humanity courses in the premed curriculum.

At semester break in his second year, Bruce stayed in Colorado to go skiing with the Presbyterian student group, so he did not come home. When his grades came, he still did not have any biology or chemistry courses. My father thought the university was all wrong in having this curriculum. Finally, in the summer, when Bruce's grades came in for his fourth semester and there were still no science courses, Bruce admitted to Dad that he had changed his major halfway through his first year and was now majoring in languages. He had changed his mind about becoming a doctor. I do not know whether Dad was more upset over Bruce's change of major or the fact that he had not told him he did it.

Bruce had taken Spanish in high school, and my mother found a student trip to Mexico for him to take during the summer between his third and fourth years in high school. He thoroughly enjoyed the trip and speaking Spanish in Mexico. During the summer after he graduated from high school, my mother arranged through a neighbor for Bruce to work for the Venezuela Gas Company in Caracas, Venezuela. Bruce lived there for two months under the eye of our neighbor's brother, the vice president of the gas company. Bruce helped create a bilingual catalog of the products sold by the gas company.

While he was in Venezuela, he learned to be quite proficient in Spanish, including the local idioms and profanity. He also learned to speak Spanish with a Venezuelan accent. Venezuelans do not pronounce the *s*'s, so it sounds very different from either school Spanish or Castilian Spanish. They say "Como eta uted?" instead of "Como esta usted?" His vocabulary was better than his fellow students, but he drove his college Spanish professor nuts with his pronunciation.

Bruce had a love of languages and a desire to travel that exceeded his desire to become a doctor, especially if it meant his return to Normal, Illinois. He did not like biology or direct responsibility for people's lives, so he made the right choice.

Chapter 19

Dad continued his love of travel. In 1957, the year I graduated from high school, an opportunity presented that he could not pass up. Illinois State Normal University celebrated its centennial year in a special way.

The geography department was very important for training teachers during that era. Every year, ISNU offered summer school classes for teachers. To renew a teaching certificate in Illinois, the applicant had to present either a master's degree or proof of at least three recent hours of graduate college courses toward a master's degree. The geography department offered a three-hour course every summer called a geography field survey.

These geography field surveys started in the 1930s as bus trips to study the geology and geography of the western states and the Rocky Mountains. After World War II, the trips began going to Europe. One year the trip would go to Scandinavia, the next would be the Mediterranean, or Germanic countries to make each year different. There were lectures and a final exam to make it a bona fide college course.

In honor of the university's centennial year, the geography department combined the two four-week summer school terms and made the course an eight-week trip around the world with eight hours of college credit. When my parents learned about the course, they immediately enrolled.

They knew the professor, Dr. Arthur W. Watterson, very well and asked if Bruce and I could take the course. Dr. Watterson thought it would be good to have some young people on the trip and approved the idea. Bruce would have completed his third year of college, so he could take the course as an upper-division transfer student. I presented a problem because I had not enrolled in college although I had been accepted to Purdue. For me to enroll in the course, I would need to have the permission of the ISNU president, Dr. Bone.

That turned out to not be much of a problem. Dr. Bone lived about one block from our house, and I mowed Dr. Bone's grass every week. When I rang the doorbell to collect my two dollars on Saturday afternoon the next week, I asked him what I needed to do to get his permission to enroll in the geography field survey. He told me that he would tell his secretary to send a memo to Dr. Watterson, authorizing my enrollment. Small towns work!

All four of us took the course. We had weeks of vaccinations, passport and visa applications, shopping for travel clothes, and selecting cameras before the trip. I took a one-semester high school course in world geography over the objections of the principal, who said it was not a college-prep course. By this time, Mom was president of the school board and overruled him.

The trip started with three days of geography lectures on campus and a group bus trip to Springfield, Illinois, for everyone to get vaccinated for yellow fever. This vaccination could only be done by a government agency and was only done once each week. The vaccine was expensive, so they wanted to get the maximum number of injections from each vial of inoculant.

The first leg of the trip was a bus trip to Chicago. We flew from Midway Airport in Chicago to JFK in New York. TWA was using the new Eero Saarinen terminal in New York. Our flight to

Shannon, Ireland, was on the first TWA Turbojet flight across the Atlantic. We had to stop in Goose Bay, Labrador, to refuel to make the hop to Shannon, Ireland. Dad told us that he had stopped to refuel there on his way home from Greenland.

There were thirty-six people on that tour including the professor, whom we all called Prof, and his wife Tony. Besides my parents and Prof and Tony, there was one other couple. The third couple turned out to be rather nonsocial, so my parents did a lot with Prof and Tony. The local tour guide would often take the tour director with his wife to a special dinner, and my parents were often included. On free evenings, the two couples often went out on the town together. They became very good friends.

While they were running around with Prof and Tony, Bruce and I had a group of young friends who did the towns at night. There were several young teachers only a few years out of school and one other college student. All in all, there were seven of us who would take the local transportation to go pub hopping or just walk the parks and streets.

When we were in Ireland, the temperatures were unseasonably warm, reaching the nineties during the daytime. The shopkeepers were so proper that they would not take off their woolen coats while they worked in what was extreme heat for them.

To ward off the heat, our group of younger tour people went to a pub in the evening to drink Guinness. This was my first experience with beer, and Guinness Stout did not taste good to me. Cut "Af n Af" with porter, it was much better. When Dad found out, he objected, but Mom convinced him that we were in Europe where there is no drinking age. I would soon be in college, so it was good for me to learn to drink responsibly with the other young people. Bruce was supposed to make sure I behaved.

We toured Ireland for two days and kissed the Blarney Stone before flying to Glasgow and Edinburgh, Scotland. Dad was already a storyteller, but he kissed the stone "to get the gift of gab."

Prof made a big point of estuary formation of the Clyde River and the Firth of Forth because of the sinking coastlines of the British Isles. He said that the Chesapeake Bay was sinking the same way. We attended the Tattoo at Edinburgh Castle to watch three drum and bagpipe bands compete. On Sunday we attended a Scottish Presbyterian Church. The minister had such a thick accent that we could not understand him. Dad thought he rolled his r's more than the Irish minister of the Baptist Church in Normal.

In Edinburgh, our young group found a dance hall. Everyone was doing the foxtrot and moving relentlessly around the dance floor. We danced with the young people there and learned that the crowd on the dance floor moved at a uniform rate around the floor, so if you slowed down or tried to change direction, you were bumped into by the people behind. We met some nice people, drank a few beers with them, and had a fun evening.

The course was organized to have a lecture every other night for a total of about thirty lectures. This did not work out very well because of the Israeli-Egyptian war that year. The trip was originally designed to include five days in Egypt to see the temples in the Aswan area that would soon be flooded by the lake created by the Aswan Dam. Construction was just beginning on the high dam in southern Egypt.

Those five days were cancelled because of the war. The two ends of the trip were moved toward the middle to fill the gap. Rebooking the trip at the last minute meant that the group was often split between two or three hotels, making it difficult for the group to assemble for lectures after dinner. Because of this, there were only eight lectures in the sixty-four-day trip.

From Edinburgh, we took a bus the length of England to London and saw lots of lorries full of woolies (trucks full of sheep) in the English countryside. We toured London and Stratford-upon-Avon before flying to Bergen, Norway, for midsummer's night.

The Norwegians built wood fires on the hillsides to celebrate midsummer's night. White smoke was everywhere. From Bergen, we took a boat trip up the fjord and boarded a train at Flam before going "over the top" of Norway by rail to Oslo, Sweden. There was snow on the ground between the frozen lakes in the mountains.

On the fjord cruise, we stopped at a village to discharge and pick up local passengers. People on the dock were selling fresh strawberries. Dad was particularly fond of strawberries, so he got off the boat to buy some berries. When he tried to reboard, he had left his ticket on board, so they stopped him. We were watching from the top deck and managed to wave and shout to convince the ticket taker that he belonged on the ship. He shared two big boxes of berries with the whole tour group.

While we were in Oslo, most of the tour group took an optional nighttime flight north to see the sun at midnight. My father had lived through the midnight sun for two summers and wanted us to see it. We flew over snowcapped mountains in northern Norway that were bathed in bright sunlight at about 1:00 a.m. before turning around to fly back to Oslo. We toured the city and visited the Winter Olympics site.

Dad had talked with Bob Bartlett about Nansen and the *Fram* and was excited to see the ship. He was impressed with the *Fram* ice ship that had been restored and was exhibited at the Fram Museum. Dad showed me the huge beams that reinforced the bow of the ship.

I did not read the full report of Nansen's Arctic voyage in the *Fram* until years later.

From Oslo, we flew to the sparkling clean city of Stockholm. The beautifully maintained Swedish square-rigged training ship, *Auf Chapman*, was moored at the waterfront. It was the first time we had seen a square-rigged ship up close.

Then it was on to Copenhagen to see the Little Mermaid in Tivoli Gardens, the neatest amusement park we had ever seen. We toured the Tuborg and Carlsberg breweries where Dad let me sample the products since we were in Europe, where there was no drinking age. By this time, I think Dad neither objected to, nor approved, my drinking "a (1) beer." For me, these Danish beers were much better than Guinness.

Busing through the Low Countries, we saw the dikes and visited Marken Island where the people were so inbred that they were myopic and some did not appear to be too bright. We went on to Paris to see the Eifel Tower and the Louvre Museum. We strolled the "Left Bank" to see the bookstalls and the men selling "dirty postcards." That evening, our young group visited Place Pigalle to watch the prostitutes roaming the street.

The whole group went on the nightclub bus tour to see the tango dancers. We sat on bleachers and were served "champagne" that my mom said was just carbonated cheap white wine. The next day, we went to see the cathedrals at Chartres and Reims and visited the Caves of Möet and Chandon to sample real champagne. It tasted musty, like the cave in which it was aged. I thought that they were foisting off the bad stuff on the tourists, but Dad told me it was the really good stuff.

Prof lectured one evening on the reasons major cities, like Paris, were located on rivers with large valleys and how the Paris basin was ideal for a major city.

We took the high-speed TGV train to Geneva, where we toured the UN headquarters of UNESCO and saw Jet d'Eau, the four-hundred-sixty-foot-high fountain of water, and then drove past John Calvin's Church.

From Geneva, we took the lake steamer to Montreux where we visited the Chateau de Chillon, the castle that inspired Lord Byron to write *The Prisoner of Chillon*. From there, we took a very modern Swiss train to Interlaken. We toured central Switzerland by Postes Bus with a horn that played the first four notes of the William Tell Overture to establish the right-of-way on hairpin turns. The Alps were full of cowbells and glaciers.

Then on to Munich, where we saw the famous town hall clock and visited the Hofbrau House. The tour continued through the Tyrol on the way to Salzburg with its mountain top castle and Vienna with Schonbrunn Palace.

From Vienna, we flew to Rome to tour the Forum and Catacombs and attend a production of Carmen at the Baths of Caracalla. One man in our group was delighted because Carmen was his favorite opera. In Rome's production of Carmen, they had real horse-drawn carriages onstage. We drank *café caldo* (hot coffee) in little glass bottles with straws during intermission. Our opera fan of the group, Jim, fell asleep during the third act. The applause awakened him at the end of the act. He stood up and started to put his jacket on to leave. We had to tell him that the opera was not over and there was a fourth act. We missed by one night the production of *Aida* with real elephants onstage during the triumphal march.

We took a bus to Florence to see the statue of David, the Duomo, the Uffizi museum, and the renaissance churches. Prof gave a lecture on the city states and the formation of modern Italy. We visited some of the small hill towns and ate good food and drank red wine.

From Italy, we flew to Athens to see the Parthenon and other Greek ruins. Our hotel was on the edge of town. The chef of the hotel restaurant had spent time in the United States and was delighted to have a group of Americans for whom he could cook American food. The whole group rebelled on our second night and went to an alfresco restaurant in the neighborhood for Greek food.

We went from Athens to Istanbul to see the grand bazaar and magnificent Mosques. We ate lunch along the Bosporus where we watched men manually unloading a barge full of huge bags of grain. The men would bend over to put a huge sack (we speculated that it weighed one hundred pounds) on their backs and walk from the barge to the wharf across a plank about a foot wide. After they dumped the sack on a pile, they trudged back to the barge for another sack. Dad told me that I needed to succeed in college to avoid that type of work.

Our young group went up to the rooftop bar of the Hilton Hotel after dinner to watch belly dancers and have a few drinks. For some reason that I do not remember, we were drinking screwdrivers. Both Bruce and I got very sick that night and had trouble making the flight to Beirut the next day. My parents thought we had stomach flu. (From bad orange juice?)

We were still sick the next day and missed the trip to the ancient ruins of the Beqaa Valley. Dad was very enthusiastic about the preserved state of the ruins in the valley when they returned. Wars since then have destroyed most of the ruins.

The next day, Bruce and I went on an optional trip to Damascus with four others from our group in two taxis. It took us an hour to clear the border going into Syria and an hour and a half to get back out of Syria that afternoon. Apparently, Syrian customs were checking our passport names for any Jewish connections. We saw Damascus from the windows of our cabs. It looked like all the other crowded dirty Arab cities.

Bruce and I bought Arab head scarves and wore them back to Beirut. When we pulled up at the hotel two hours late, Dad saw the head scarves through the cab window and thought that we had the police with us because we had gotten in trouble with the law.

We did not go to Israel on that trip because of the recent war and the high feelings on both sides. The common knowledge was that you could not get into Israel if you had a stamp in your passport from an Arab country and vice versa.

We did go to Jerusalem, Jordan. In 1957, Jerusalem was divided into two cities by a strip of no-man's-land that was patrolled by the UN. Our hotel overlooked the no-man's-land where we could see white jeeps with UN painted on the top patrolling the roads along walls on both sides of the strip. Gates were open during the day for people to walk across the strip on fenced pathways. We were told that there were minefields between the designated walkways.

From the hotel dining room, we could see the Israeli side of Jerusalem. I tried to take a photo of the view, but a tourist policeman who was stationed in the dining room ran over to me demanding that I not take the picture. He told me he would take the film from my camera if I did. When I asked why, he told me that what I saw (Israel) did not exist, therefore there was nothing to see or photograph. I took the picture while sitting at a table by the window and hiding the camera.

We were fascinated by the stories told by the guides about the exact times and dates that cannons were fired across the strip and the returned fire. They had the times down to the minute. There were large tent cities at the edge of town with sixteen-foot-high chain-link fences topped with barbed wire where the Palestinian refugees lived. The refugees had not assimilated into the Jordan people in the ten years since Palestine became Israel.

Our thirty-six-member group was too large for most of the Air Jordan planes, so we had to fly earlier than expected for our flight to the Cairo Airport to connect with a flight to Bombay. They had to substitute a larger aircraft and change the schedule.

Before the plane could take off, a flock of sheep had to be cleared from the runway. A road crossed the runway, and the flock was passing through.

The airport was very near the Israeli border, and the prevailing wind in Jerusalem was from the west, out of Israel. We took off into the wind. Once the wheels were literally just off the ground, the plane banked hard to the left to avoid flying over Israel. We had to fly all around the southern tip of Israel and back northwest to Cairo to avoid Israeli airspace. The runways at the Cairo airport were patched, and there were carters in the ground around them from the bombing during the war several months before.

We were supposed to land in Cairo at 6:00 p.m., but, because of the early flight, we arrived at noon. Our flight to Bombay was to leave at midnight. The Cairo Airport was not air-conditioned that July and we did not have visas for Egypt, so we were supposed to stay in the hot airport for twelve hours.

Prof was an experienced tour guide. He went over to the money-changing office and exchanged some money. Then he walked around the customs area and talked with each of the customs officers. He would reach in his pocket and then shake hands with each officer. After a short discussion with the chief officer, he came to the waiting hall and told us all to grab our carry-on luggage and follow him. He led us out through the customs hall to a line of taxis. We all climbed into the taxis and soon we were off across country.

After a short ride, we arrived near the pyramids and the Sphinx. The parking area was over a hundred yards from the pyramids, but there was a line of camels and horses. Prof told us to pick a camel or horse for the ride to the pyramids.

Our family all climbed onto the camels that were lying on the ground. At the command of the driver, the camel stood. This involved unfolding the back legs, throwing the rider forward, then unfolding the front legs, throwing the rider backward. There were two steps to unfolding the front and back legs, so it was hard to stay in the camel saddle, but we all managed. It seemed that I was ten feet off the ground when the camel was fully standing.

My driver immediately looked up at me and said, "Baksheesh?"

I did not have any Egyptian money, so I shrugged and held my hands out, palm up, the universal sign for having no money. The driver then hit the camel on the back of the neck with a long stick. The camel leapt forward and set off at a gallop. There were no reins and no pommel on the saddle. I grabbed the front edge of the saddle and held on for dear life. The camel stopped running after about fifty yards.

The driver ran up and put up his hand and said, "Now baksheesh?"

I dug into my pocket and gave him the two Jordanian coins that I had left.

He pocketed the coins and reached up again, saying, "More baksheesh, I have four children."

I made the "no money" gesture again. The remainder of the ride was uneventful. Mom and Dad and Bruce rode camels, but did not have that experience.

From the pyramids we went to a shopping area to buy souvenirs and then to the brand-new Russian-built Cairo Hilton to rest in the lobby. Prof made arrangements for dinner at a restaurant about two blocks from the hotel. The restaurant had a belly dancer show with Arab music that lasted through the evening. We were bused back to the airport in time for our flight to Bombay. For "not being in Egypt," we had hit the highlights.

We landed in Bombay between monsoons. The tarmac was covered with big puddles and there were dark clouds overhead, but it was not raining. Bombay was just a plane change on the way to Delhi. Delhi was a hot, dry, dirty sprawling city with many more bicycles than cars.

Our hotel had been built for a United Nations conference and was very nice. Because of the heat, the Indians all took siestas in the early afternoon. I recall lying in bed watching the salamanders run up and down the walls and across the ceiling of our room.

Dad and Mom joined the local tour director with Prof and Tony for dinner. They sat on the floor and ate an assortment of exotic often spicy foods with their fingers. There were no forks or spoons. It was a very new experience for both couples.

The local tour director arranged for the finance minister of India to speak to us one evening. He explained that when India won their independence from the British, the new parliament was reluctant to do any deficit financing. The tax revenues were too low for any large investments, so the government had let the industrial infrastructure, left by the British, deteriorate and break down. The examples he gave were that railroads could hardly run and the steel mills were operating well below capacity. This was crippling the Indian economy, so poverty was rampant.

We took a bus to Agra, leaving at 4:00 a.m. to avoid the heat of the day. We stopped in a village along the way where women were doing laundry in reddish-brown water in a pond where water buffalo stood in the water.

There was a man plowing a field with a wooden one-bottom plow that was pulled by a Brahma cow. He stopped for us to take his picture. When Dad offered to send him his picture, he was very pleased, but could not give us an address to which to send it. Our guide and translator explained that he had never received a letter.

There were three flocks of buzzards at separate places in the field. The farmer told us that three cows had died and their carcasses had attracted the buzzards.

When we went back to the bus that was parked next to the pond, some of our companions took pictures of the women washing the clothes. Several of the women took offense to being photographed, so they started yelling and throwing rocks. We escaped with only one broken window and a few dents on the bus. Obviously, the women had a different opinion of photography from the man plowing the field.

The main reason for going to Agra was to see the Taj Mahal. There is a long reflecting pool with gardens on either side along the approach to the Taj. There were three men mowing the grass in the garden. One was steering a fifteen-inch-wide reel lawnmower, one was driving the Brahma cow that was pulling the mower, and the third man was directing the activity. India was trying for full employment.

The Taj is made of white marble that is inlaid with semiprecious stones in ornate patterns. The whiteness is dazzling in the midday sun; it glowed in the moonlight. It was built in memory of the ruler's wife. We were told that he would have built a similar temple in black marble across the river with the bridge between them if the people had not risen against him for his extravagance.

Every time we left our hotel, there were several men with snakes, cobras and pythons, waiting at the gate. They wanted to drape the snakes around the tourists and take pictures of them. Dad, always the good sport, went along with them and had several snakes draped over his shoulders and around his neck. We all took his picture.

In the marketplace that night, there was a boy about twelve years old who was charming a cobra in a basket. After several minutes of the cobra waving back and forth, the cobra lay down in the basket. The boy grabbed the lid of the basket and held it out for tips as he went around the crowd.

When he was about halfway around the crowd, the snake came out of the basket and started slithering across the pavement. Everyone yelled at the boy, who ran over to pick up the cobra and hung it over his shoulders and around his neck. Then he returned to the crowd with the basket lid for more tips. Everyone ran away from him because of the snake, so he did not get any more tips. We were told later that all the cobras that were allowed within the city had been detoxified and were harmless.

I bought a travel chess set with black-and-white ivory chess pieces that pegged onto the wood and ivory chessboard box. I asked Dad to teach me to play chess, but he said that it had been so long since he had taken the time to play chess that he did not remember the moves of the different pieces. Our local guide taught me the basic moves but proceeded to beat me several times. Dad preferred to play cribbage.

When we flew over Calcutta and the Ganges River on the way to Bangkok, we could see that everything was flooded from the monsoons, so we could not have visited Calcutta.

The plane landed in Bangkok where we stayed in the very posh Erawan House Hotel. We saw the Emerald Buddha, which was carved from a single huge emerald. We were impressed by the beautiful temple towers that were surfaced with broken china. They were very colorful, but did not look too functional as temples.

The floating market with shallow canoes full of beautifully prepared produce floating in very dirty, foul-smelling water was a study in contrasts. Strings of ebony logs were being floated down the river. Ebony is so heavy that it had to be tied to other logs to keep it from sinking.

We flew over most of Southeast Asia and lots of water to land in Hong Kong. We had to change our schedule again because there was a shortage of pilots who could land a plane the size we needed in Hong Kong. The runway was short and ended with both ends in the water. As we landed, I thought that the masts of the sampans docked near the end of the runway would come up through the wings because we were flying so low over the water to be able to land at the very end of the runway.

Hong Kong was a bustling city full of rickshaws. We stayed in Kowloon, in the brand-new Peninsula Hotel Annex, across the side street from the main hotel. Dad said the hotel was so new that the paint was not dry on the seat of the commode in their room. When we crossed the street to go for dinner, the rickshaw boys would run up to us and say, "Yunior, Yump in lickshaw, go for lide! I take you meet my sister, she velly nice."

We took a day excursion to the island of Hong Kong to visit Tiger Balm Gardens, named after Tiger Balm, which is a salve that the

Chinese used to cure anything involving muscles, skin, headaches, abdominal gas, sore throats among other illnesses. From the location of the garden, high on the mountain, we could see the tops of the city buildings. They looked rough and cluttered. We learned that they were covered by cardboard villages where the homeless refugees lived. People were pouring out of China into British Hong Kong, but there was nowhere for them to live.

Dad took Bruce and me to a Hong Kong tailor shop. We were all measured for suits and sport coats. The next day, the tailor came to the hotel with partially made clothes for the first fitting. The clothes were all finished and delivered the next morning before we left Hong Kong. When I tried on the suits at home, I discovered that the styles were cut differently from the current American styles, so they looked strange.

We took an overnight ferry to Macao, Portuguese Crown Colony, known for its gambling. We watched a game being played that had three dice in a covered glass dome. The covered dome was shaken and placed on a table. Bets were placed for about fifteen minutes before the cover was removed from the glass dome to read the dice and determine the winners.

We visited a fireworks factory where small children, three to five years old, were crimping the ends of paper rolls to make firecrackers. They were working for food. After they crimped several packets of tubes, they would be given something to eat. Dad pointed out to one of the supervisors that several of these children had patches of impetigo and looked undernourished. The manager told Dad it was none of his business.

There was a village on the outskirts of Macao that was surrounded by gardens. The workers were carrying large watering cans on yokes on their shoulders while running through the fields to water the plants. They filled the cans at a pond in the middle of the fields. We could tell by the smell that the gardens were fertilized with "night soil." Years later, in medical school, I learned that this practice was the reason for so many intestinal parasites in that part of the world.

We could see the Chinese border from the village, and several of us decided to walk over to get a closer look. When we got about fifty yards from the gate and guardhouse, two soldiers came to attention and lowered their automatic rifles to firing position. We decided to turn around and go back to the village.

We stayed in the Frank Lloyd Wright–designed Imperial Hotel in Tokyo. It was supposed to be the first hotel in Japan that was earthquake proof. The ceilings were only about six feet four inches high, so the building was so short that an earthquake would not shake it down. Tokyo was a very crowded city full of hurrying people.

We took the bullet train from Tokyo to Kyoto. The conductor came through the train and told Prof that the train would be thirty seconds late arriving in Kyoto. To make up the time, the train would only stay in the station for thirty seconds rather than the scheduled sixty seconds.

There were thirty-six people in our group to get off at the station. Some were older ladies who did not move very fast. Bruce and I and the other two young men on the trip were recruited to stack the luggage in the seats by the operable windows on the side of the train toward the platform. Dad made sure that everyone else was lined up in the aisle and moved toward the doors. He was in charge of shepherding half of the people off of one end of the train car. Prof took the other end.

As soon as we reached the platform, we started putting suitcases out the open windows onto the platform, even before the train stopped. When the last suitcase was out the window, we climbed out the window and the train started to move. We had to gather up the suitcases from the length of the platform.

We toured Shinto shrines and the Golden Pagoda in Kyoto and stayed in a hotel with huge gardens that were all various shades of green. Since none of the younger group could speak Japanese, we decided to go to the hotel bar to have a drink after dinner rather than into town.

One of the old maid schoolteachers came into the bar to get bottled water to brush her teeth. She saw our group and came over to talk with us. Actually, she came to lecture us. She said that we young "whippersnappers" should be in our rooms studying. We should not have been running around at night partying throughout the trip. This trip was a college course, and there would be an exam. Because we had not stayed in at night to study, we would not get good grades like she would.

Prof decided to give the final exam in Kyoto because the group was splitting up in Hawaii. He commandeered the main dining room after dinner and passed out the exams. There were ten essay questions based on the lectures in Normal and the eight on the trip.

Bruce and I had attended all the lectures so it was not much of a challenge to regurgitate what he had said. My dad had not paid attention to the lectures and struggled some with the exam although nothing was at stake for him. My mom did not even try to answer the questions. She launched into a memoir of the trip, mostly about the things she and Dad had done with Prof and Tony. Each question triggered a memory of something on the trip, so she wrote as long as most of the exam takers and turned in her paper. Prof took the exams home to grade.

From Kyoto, we took the train to Osaka to board a plane to fly home through Hawaii. We stopped at Midway to refuel the Super G

Constellation and have breakfast. The four engines of the Super G were not synchronized, so they were slightly out of phase and made a cyclic vibration for the eight-hour duration of each leg of the flight. We crossed the international date line between Midway and Hawaii. The course tour was scheduled to overnight in Hawaii to change planes and fly home. Several of the travelers, including our family, stayed for four nights at the Moana Hotel in Honolulu.

Mom and Dad had been in Hawaii before for a medical meeting and wanted Bruce and me to see Oahu. After visits to Pearl Harbor and Honolulu and the drive around the island to the pineapple fields, Dad bought a surfing lesson for Bruce and me by one of the native surfers. After two hours of lying on surfboards trying to catch waves, we both had painful sunburns on our backs.

Sitting for eight hours on the plane to San Francisco that night was miserably painful. The connection in Los Angeles took us to Chicago on the first day that O'Hare Airport opened in August 1957. We had to walk under scaffolding and tarpaulins to get out of the airport, which was still being painted. For us, the trip had gone around the world in sixty-eight days. Dad talked about that trip for the rest of his life.

My parents had become such good friends with Prof and Tony that we ate Thanksgiving dinner with them that fall. I knew that our whole family had received grades of A for the course. I wondered if Prof had given everyone As. Dad asked him, as we were finishing dessert, how the grades ranged. Prof explained that graduate courses were graded from A to C with C being failing in grad school. He told Dad that everyone in our course had gotten As and Bs, but no Cs. I asked him how he decided who got the As and Bs. He told me that it was mostly test scores, but some of the people did not get as much out of the trip as we did. When I told him about the lady bawling us out for running around, he told me that he thought our young group got more out of the trip than anyone else. We had seen the towns up close and met the people.

Mom asked him about her exam. He told us that her exam was about halfway through the stack. He was tired of reading the same old answers by that time, so he kicked back in his chair, put his feet on his desk, and read her stories. He thoroughly enjoyed them and decided that she had learned a lot about the world and derived what she wanted from the trip, so he gave it an A.

Dad had bought a new Retina IIIC Kodak camera for the trip. He liked it so much that he gave one to Bruce and one to me. He bought thirty-six rolls of film with thirty-six exposures per roll for himself and gave Bruce and me each twenty-five rolls of thirty-six shots. He admonished us throughout the trip not to waste film because it might be hard to find in the Far East. He ran out of his thirty-six rolls in Bangkok and tried to borrow film from us. We had not hoarded our film to give it to him, so we managed to always have our extra film in our suitcases. He had to buy film along the way.

The film he bought abroad came with a small can and a tagged pouch to send the exposed film to Kodak for prepaid developing. Bruce and I took our film with Dad's first thirty-six rolls to the photo shop in Normal for developing and paid for it when we picked up the slides. Dad got the rest of his pictures back in the mail.

One of the women on the trip had purchased a new camera on the day before we started. She had not had a chance to run a roll of film through the camera to see how it worked. When her film came back from processing, it was all blank. She had not realized that she needed to cock the shutter on the lens before every picture. She was devastated. She called Prof to tell him what happened. Prof sent a letter to everyone who had been on the trip to appeal for second-best shots, or what my dad called culls. Dad sent her a big bundle of slides. She was inundated with slides from the other travelers and put together her own set of slides from the culls. Prof said that it was probably the most comprehensive set of the whole group.

Chapter 20

Dad was very disappointed by the fact that Bruce had decided not to become a doctor, but may have been more upset by the fact that he had hidden his decision. He had really wanted Bruce to follow him in his profession. My mother blamed Dad for pressuring Bruce into saying he wanted to become a doctor and pushing him into premed. They argued a lot about this. I think they decided not to put any pressure on me about my career choice or the choice of a college.

Everyone in my math and science classes was planning to become an engineer or major in math or chemistry. Bruce and I were the only students in our high school who were sons of a doctor. Both of my parents encouraged me to follow my choice of engineering. I did enjoy industrial drawing, but I did not want to work at a drawing board all my life. I wanted to play a role in conquering space.

During the summer between my junior and senior years in high school, we went on a combination school-visiting trip and vacation. The Longs, Lee, Sugar, and Molly went with us in Dad's car. Molly was a year older than me. Bruce did not go.

We skipped the University of Illinois because it was too close to home. The first stop was Purdue University in West Lafayette, Indiana. Purdue had a good engineering school, and all the astronauts had trained there. Purdue had lots of four-story red brick buildings and new dormitories. We were favorably impressed.

The next stop was to visit Carnegie Institute of Technology in Pittsburgh, Pennsylvania. Dad was used to driving in cities with rectangular grids of streets, and Pittsburgh was anything but that. We found the Oakland section of Pittsburgh and drove around the area where Carnegie Tech was shown on the map. We circled the Cathedral of Learning of the University of Pittsburgh several times and got lost in Schenley Park, but we could not find Carnegie Tech. Dad told me that I did not want to go to school in a dirty industrial city like Pittsburgh anyway, so we headed for central New York State to see Cornell.

We made it to Ithaca, New York, and followed signs to Cornell, which was on top of a hill, overlooking Lake Cayuga. One of the pamphlets we picked up explained that the engineering and agriculture schools were run by the state of New York and the rest of the school was a private university. We were told that the engineering school did not like to take out-of-state students. Dad said that upstate New York had lots of ice and snow in the winter, so I would not like it there. He said, "If you are not careful, you could slip on the ice, fall on your butt, and slide all the way down the hill and into the lake." We should press on to Boston and MIT.

When we were about fifty miles out of Boston, Dad and Lee got into a discussion about who would drive in Boston. Dad had been there for meetings and was sure he would get lost or he might have an accident because everyone in Boston drove like they were crazy. Dad told me that MIT and Harvard were full of effete eastern snobs and I would not get along well with them, so we should skip MIT and head for Maine for our vacation. We went from Maine to Quebec City and up the St. Lawrence to Montreal and back to Normal.

Dad wanted me to go to the University of Illinois, but I decided on Purdue University because they had a degree in engineering sciences.

This curriculum had courses in math, physics, chemistry, and all fields of engineering. It supposedly prepared the elite engineers to lead the way. Many of the courses did not use numbers, but used letters to demonstrate the theory and deemphasize the precision of numbers. The goal was to be able to understand and supervise engineering, not do it. At first, I did not realize that it was a pre-master's degree preparation. I think it was in my junior year when I realized that graduates were supposed to get a master's degree in management or economics or go to law school to get to the management level of industry.

I did well at Purdue. When I made all As the first semester, I was very excited. I called home to tell my parents that I was one of the sixteen students at Purdue who made straight As. Mom answered the phone because Dad was making house calls. I told her my good news and expected some congratulations and praise, but all Mom said was, "Good, that's what we expected. See if you can do it again next term."

On the first day of classes the next term, I reported to my English Composition course and was greeted by Mr. Kidd. He told us that he was "the Captain." He graded with a hard pencil and did not give a grade above a C. If anyone deserved a grade higher than a C, they would have tested out of English 101 and been in 103. I decided that I had no chance of getting straight As, so I might as well relax on the grades and have some fun in college.

That term was fraternity rush for students who lived in the dormitories the first year. I planned to go through rush and join a fraternity. There was an Acacia chapter at Purdue. Since my father was an Acacian at Missouri U and my brother was in Acacia at U of Colorado, I decided to include Acacia in the fraternities that I rushed.

It finally came down to a decision between Delta Tau Delta and Acacia. The Delts had a fairly new house and a Rah! Rah! group of guys. The Acacians were a serious but fun-loving group who had several upper-class members who were campus leaders and were very impressive. I agonized over this for a few days after I received bids from both houses. I finally decided to go family and joined Acacia.

When I told my parents, I was surprised by the enthusiasm from my father. He told me that he had hoped that I would pledge Acacia, but was afraid to push me that way for fear that it might push me away. Was this the shadow of Bruce?

I continued to do well at Purdue, making the honor roll, but no more straight As. I was sitting in a fluid dynamics course on the Friday afternoon before homecoming weekend during my fifth term. At the end of the class, the instructor assigned a big group of problems to solve before the class on Monday. I do not think the professor knew that it was homecoming weekend. The entire class let out a collective groan at the size of the assignment.

The professor turned to the class and gave us a lecture about how we should be "gung ho to run home and tackle these problems." He elaborated that as engineers, this is what we would be doing for the rest of our lives. If we did not have the desire to go solve these problems, we should look for another profession.

I had been raised by parents who were devoted to doing things to help others. By this time, I was vice president of Acacia and liked being part of administration and helping my fraternity brothers in school and house activities. The idea of working with impersonal engineering problems for the rest of my life was becoming unattractive.

Because of my admiration for my father, who was always trying to make life better for someone, I thought about becoming a doctor. That would involve switching to premed studies, possibly changing universities, possibly adding a year or more in college, and then four years of medical school, an internship, and a maybe a residency for three or more years. The Korean War was still going on, and the draft was very possible after graduation. This meant nine or ten years of more school and military time.

I thought about it for several days. I checked the Purdue catalog and discovered that there was a premed curriculum. I contacted Dr. James, the premed adviser and talked to him about transferring. He told me that I already had many of the required courses for medical school admission and could finish the curriculum in three more semesters. It would require a transfer from engineering school to the science school, but that was easy.

I went back to the fraternity house and called home. Dad was home so they were both on the line. I told them I was thinking about changing my major, and they immediately chimed in that I was a bit late in college to be thinking about that. I told them that I had done some research and knew that I could complete the new major in the same time as engineering. I told them that I wanted to switch to premed and become a doctor. It took my father about three seconds to say that the change would be great. I could come back to Normal and join him in practice after my training.

My parents were very generous in supporting Bruce and me through school. They told us that they would finance us as far as we wanted to go in school as long as we did not get married. Dad was proud of having worked his way through school, but did not want us to have to give up all that he had given up to be able to go to college.

They had set up trust funds for Bruce and me when Bruce started college. These were ten-year irrevocable trusts that were funded by Pearl Brewery stock. Since we both went to state schools, the $3,000 plus per year from these trusts was sufficient for our school expenses. I knew that medical school would probably be more expensive. Dad agreed to pay my tuition to medical school.

Remembering the "stay single" part of the educational backing, I decided to take advantage of the euphoric atmosphere to bring this up. I did not have any prospects for marriage at that time, but told them that I was not sure that I wanted to stay single until I finished medical school so I asked if they would still support me if I were married. My dad was on a high at that point and said that they would not expect me to stay single after I graduated from premed.

I went back to see Dr. James on Monday to arrange for the transfer. He went to work while I was in his office trying to get me into the courses I needed for premed. He knew that I would need organic chemistry and that many premed students had to take it twice to pass it so I should take it as soon as possible.

He called the chemistry department and learned that the premed-level biochemistry course was full for the next semester. He told me not to worry. All I needed was three hours of biochemistry on my application to medical school. The course number would not matter. He called the chemistry department back and enrolled me in a three-hour home economics biochemistry course.

Then we ran into a problem. There was a graduation requirement in the science school that had not been required in engineering. For several years, the science school had required a course called General Studies. It was a four-semester integrated curriculum combining history, economics, humanities, and government. The course could only be started in the fall semester.

The catalog said that with the permission of the dean, four humanities courses could be substituted for the GS course. I had taken one philosophy course while I was in engineering so I only needed three more humanities courses, which I could fit into my schedule with one course each semester.

I made an appointment with Dean Ayers and presented my case. I thought it would be straightforward and the substitution would allow me to graduate on time. The dean told me that he had helped design the GS series and thought that every student that graduated from Purdue should take all four semesters, not just the students enrolled in the science school, the only school that had this requirement. He said that I should begin the GS sequence in the fall semester of my fourth year and then come back for a fifth year to take the third and fourth semesters of GS along with some electives to fill my time. I could graduate in five years. I pleaded about the number of years of school, college plus medical school, plus internship and residency and then military ahead of me, but to no avail. He was intent on making me take the GS courses.

In engineering, I had been taking twenty-two to twenty-four credit hours every semester and would have a heavy load to finish the premed curriculum. I knew that Purdue had a rule about a maximum number of hours a student could accumulate without graduating. Once that number was reached, the student would not be allowed to continue in school. I would have to petition the school to get permission to reenroll to take the required courses to graduate.

I asked the dean if he could guarantee that I would be able to enroll for the fifth year with the many hours I would have completed by then. He looked me straight in the eye and told me that he could never guarantee anything like that. I asked him how he could require me to arrange my curriculum to add a year in school but not reassure me that I could actually do it. He said I would have to do it and take my chances.

When I told my parents about the predicament, my father told me that college graduation was not a requirement for medical school admission as long as I had completed the required courses and had good grades. At that point, I thought "forget graduation and do the required courses for medical school." Actually, I probably thought, "Screw Purdue. If they won't let me graduate, I will never give them a dime." I haven't.

The home economics biochemistry course was a snap. The textbook was in an 8 × 10 format, less than a half inch thick, with lots of pictures and diagrams of molecules. It dealt with things like the changes of the temperature at which water boiled when salt or antifreeze was added, telling alcohols from aldehydes and why yeast rises. This course did not get into serious biochemistry like metabolism and enzymes. I got an A for three hours of biochemistry on my transcript.

My comparative anatomy course was easy once we figured out that the professor arranged the answer letters for the multiple-choice questions so that they spelled a genus or species in the answer column when all the answers were correct. That made his exam grading easier for him. We had to learn enough to get most of the answers right so that we could use the corrected spelling to get the right answers for the ones we did not know. I always allowed a few intentional errors to keep it from being obvious that I knew the system.

Physiology and embryology were more difficult, but not as hard as differential equations and the theory of probability I had taken in engineering. I had good grades and a good GPA for my applications for medical school.

My dad was excited to have me in the medical field and wanted me to go into surgery so I could come home and take over his practice. He told me that he would take me to the operating room to watch him do surgery when I came home for spring break. Unfortunately, Dr. Fruin's son, Alan, was studying premed and was home for spring break the week before Purdue's spring break. Dr. Fruin took Alan to the operating room to watch surgery. Alan passed out when he saw blood and split open his scalp when he collapsed onto the terrazzo floor. He had to be revived by the operating room staff and have stitches in his scalp. The hospital immediately made a rule that no nonmedical people would be allowed to watch surgery, so I could not watch my dad. By the time I finished my second year in medical school, he had retired so I never got to watch my father do surgery.

During my second term in premed, I asked my dad where I should apply to medical school. His first reply was Washington University. He graduated there, and he thought that they produced good doctors. He told me that Dr. Shultz, the local orthopedist, had gone to the University of Wisconsin Medical School and he was a very good doctor. I applied to both schools.

The word circulating at Purdue was not to bother to apply to Indiana University Medical School if you were from out of state. The previous year, the Indiana legislature had gone through a big argument about funding medical training for out-of-state students, so the school was not admitting anyone except Indiana residents.

I also considered Duke Medical School. The reply to my letter requesting an application form was very discouraging. They were not accepting applications from out-of-state students unless they were in the top 10 percent of their class, which I barely missed.

Washington U had a two-stage application process. Step one was a two-page form with personal and financial information plus a transcript. If you passed that level, there was a four-page application form with the last page left blank for a personal essay about why you chose to become a doctor. There were also three fill in the blanks, letters to be filled in by three professors and mailed directly to the admissions office. I took the letters to three professors who had given me As.

Two days after I delivered the letters, the chemistry professor to whom I had given the letter had a heart attack. When I heard about it, I went to see his secretary to see if he had sent the letter. She said that she did not know, and she refused to check his desk to see if it was still there. I wanted to give it to another professor if he had not done it. She refused to even check his desk, saying that she was to see to it that he did not do any work during his convalescence. I guess she thought I would try to take it to him at home.

I went back to the Acacia house and called the medical school admissions office. The secretary said that it was not a problem. She would send me another letter to give to a different professor.

While this was happening, Bruce had a flare-up of his ulcerative colitis. It was very bad, so Dad took him to the Washington University Clinics for evaluation. The doctors decided that his disease was destroying his colon, causing bleeding and dehydration, and concluded that he would only survive if his entire colon was removed. Dr. Carl Moyer, the chief of surgery, would do the operation.

My dad learned that Dr. Moyer was chairman of the admissions committee that year and told him that I was applying to medical school. I learned later that my dad would ask Dr. Moyer every day when he made rounds on Bruce if he had seen my application and whether I would be admitted.

On Saturday morning at the end of the week of my brother's surgery, my father called me at the fraternity house. He had good news. He had talked to Dr. Moyer that morning, and the doctor had said not to worry, I would be in the next class, starting in 1961. At this point, I knew that I was a legacy admission because I had just delivered the replacement letter to a professor that morning, meaning that my application was not complete. Some of my classmates were getting rejection letters, so I was glad to be in. About a month later,

I received a letter of acceptance from the University of Wisconsin, so I would have gotten into a medical school where I was not a legacy.

There is something about doctor's families having complications. On the night after the surgery, Bruce was bothered by the nasogastric tube and pulled it out. He became distended after that. This is not uncommon after abdominal surgery. An intern was sent in to replace the nasogastric tube into Bruce's stomach to relieve the distension. Bruce gagged so much during the insertion of the tube that he tore out his abdominal stitches and had be taken back to the operating room to be resutured. Bruce had no respect for interns after that and would not let them touch him.

Dad had taken Bruce to several specialists for diagnosis and treatment of his colitis. The thinking about ulcerative colitis at that time was that it was caused by stress. My father never accepted that cause and insisted that Bruce led a stress-free life because he was able to perform well in school and his home life was calm and stress free.

Several times when we were younger, Bruce called me back to his room and closed the door to tell me that he thought that our parents were going to get a divorce. They argued constantly and had shouting matches in front of us. Bruce told me that they had made provisions in their wills for us to be taken care of by the Longs. Bruce somehow equated a divorce of parents with orphaning of the children. He would tell me that we should try to stick together if we were abandoned by our parents. I never thought it was that serious, but Bruce seemed to think that it was imminent.

I also thought that Bruce felt a lot of pressure from my dad to become a physician, but could not bring himself to face Dad to admit that he did not want a career in medicine. He did not admit changing majors in college until it was too late to change back. My mother blamed my father for Bruce's illness, but he would not accept the blame. Although there were books about ulcerative colitis being a psychosomatic disease, Dad would not accept that Bruce had any stress in his life.

On her deathbed, Mom told me that she thought that Bruce had inherited his diseases from my father because she thought that Dad had rheumatoid arthritis, and she considered Bruce's diseases to be collagen vascular-related diseases.

In retrospect, I feel that Dad had osteoarthritis. He had knee pain in his forties after his skiing injury, but never got the typical changes of rheumatoid arthritis in his hands or other joints. Although he gave up surgery because of his arthritic hands, he was able to handle the small rocks he polished into jewelry until just before he died in his eighties. This is more typical of osteoarthritis than rheumatoid arthritis.

In his forties, living in California, Bruce developed an inflammatory disease of the lungs that went undiagnosed for several months. Finally, a pathologist at Yale read his slides from the Stanford University Hospital biopsy and called it an eosinophilic granulomatous giant cell vasculitis of the small arteries of the lungs, of presumed immune etiology.

Bruce's doctor had been treating him for allergies. Bruce was coming down with a cold after Christmas so the doctor decided to give him an allergy shot every week for four weeks, rather than his monthly shot. Bruce came down with the disease during the four weeks of allergy shots.

The disease I think he had is caused by overwhelming antigen to antibody reaction, creating a circulating antigen-antibody complex to which the body reacts by forming eosinophilic granulomata. My theory was that the repeated allergy shots caused an overload of his immune system and the antigen-antibody complexes then precipitated the allergic vasculitis in his lungs.

With the advent of stem cell and bone marrow transplants, this immune response has become well documented in relation to "Graft vs. Host Reaction" as seen in bone marrow transplants where the new transplanted immune system in the marrow sees the host's tissues as foreign.

I thought the way it was diagnosed and treated was badly done. They tried brush biopsies of the lung that were inconclusive. When they opened his chest to do an open-lung biopsy, they "discovered" a liter of fluid around the lungs. (When I was in medical school, the professors prided themselves in being able to detect 100 ccs of fluid in a chest by physical diagnosis without X-rays or surgically opening the chest.)

The doctors treated Bruce with steroids, which was appropriate, and managed to get him back on his feet. After that, he was declared a respiratory cripple and went on disability from his job at Bank of America.

When I learned that he was disabled and still on a high dose of daily steroids, I was concerned that he would become steroid dependent. He would have to stay on steroids the rest of his life or he would die. I discussed this with Dad, and he asked me to intervene.

I convinced Bruce, with help from Dad, to come to Galveston for a second opinion. His doctor fought this, but Bruce came. I asked Dr. James Guckian, one of the best diagnosticians at UTMB, to work him up. Jim learned that he had 95 percent of his pulmonary function, which meant that he was no longer breathing disabled. All of his blood work showed that the disease process was over or dormant. Jim decreased his steroids to taking them every other day so that his adrenal glands could continue to make steroids on the off days. If his adrenals could be made to produce steroids, he could eventually be weaned from steroid treatment and live without them.

Bruce went back to California where his doctor told him that we were all wrong and put him back on everyday steroids. When I argued with Bruce about this, he said that his doctor pointed out to him that he felt tired on the off days during every other day dosing, proving that he needed the steroids. I knew that this tiredness was normal for someone coming off every day treatment and the tiredness was the stimulus for his own adrenals to make steroids. Bruce made the excuse that his doctor was a social friend, so he did not want to fight with his doctor. Dad backed me on this problem of steroid dependence, but Bruce went with his doctor.

Several months after he went back to everyday dosage, he fell while getting off a Nautilus machine at the Stanford Gym and broke his arm. This was related to the steroids, which are known to weaken bones when taken for an extended time. By this time, he was steroid dependent so it took a long time for his bones to heal while he continued his steroids every day. Had he been on alternate-day steroids, his own adrenal glands would have begun making steroids again and he could have been weaned off the medications before his bones had deteriorated.

But I digress. After Bruce had his colon removed, he lived at home and decided to enroll in the University of Illinois graduate school to take classes in business and marketing. He commuted the fifty miles from Normal to University of Illinois in Urbana. While he was doing this, he met Judy Wasson. Judy was a year behind me in high school. She was very talented in piano and organ and was substitute organist at the Bloomington Baptist Church. She had been my accompanist during high school when I played marimba solos. Bruce was away at the University of Colorado at that time and did not know Judy. Mom had known Judy longer than Bruce and liked her when she worked with me.

CHAPTER 21

Early in my senior year, I represented Acacia Fraternity at an organizational meeting of the Young Republicans for Nixon at Purdue. When the moderator asked for a volunteer for precinct chairman for the sororities, Letha Foss stood up and volunteered. I thought she was very attractive and had the right politics so I wrote down her name. She was a Phi Mu, and my "little brother" in the fraternity, Bill, was pinned to Susie, a Phi Mu. When I returned to the fraternity that night, Bill and Susie were sitting in front of the fireplace. I asked Susie to fix me up with Letha. Susie objected that Letha was not my type.

I persisted, and Susie arranged for a triple date to go out for pork tenderloins and root beer at the Tri Chi (XXX) drive in. Letha was dating another student whom I did not know. I kept making dates with her to study or meet her before sorority hours for a snack. Eventually, I had her mortarboard date book filled up.

We agreed to meet after the All-Greek Dog Show that was sponsored by the Phi Mu Sorority. We went for a long ride in the country and talked for hours. We discovered that we had many commonalities in high school and college accomplishments. She did not tell me that she had just accepted the other man's fraternity pin.

Letha accepted my fraternity pin in October of my senior year. Shortly after that, Susie told me that Letha had given the other man's pin back. We dated a lot and were talking about getting engaged in the spring.

Letha came down with mononucleosis. She was very ill, so she was admitted to the Purdue infirmary. They suspected mono but had to wait until Friday for the diagnostic test. Every Friday, they drew blood from a sheep at the Purdue Agriculture School Farm to run the sheep red cell agglutination test for mono. The test was positive.

Letha had been scheduled to take the Miller analogies test at Illinois State Normal University in Normal on Saturday. The Miller analogies test was a requirement for application to psychology graduate school. That weekend was the last date the exam was offered before graduate school applications were due. We had planned to drive to Normal on Friday night so she could take the exam and spend the weekend at my home.

I called the doctor at the infirmary on Friday night to see if I could take her out of the infirmary so she could take the exam. The doctor was reluctant to release her from the infirmary until I explained that my father was a doctor who could care for her until she was ready to return to school.

The doctor jumped at the chance to get a patient with infectious mononucleosis out of the infirmary and into another doctor's hands. I assured him that I had my mother's Mercedes at school and it had reclining leather seats. I would bring several blankets to keep her warm during the trip. He agreed to release her to me and to my father's care. I picked her up Saturday morning at the infirmary and drove the hundred and fifteen miles to Normal. She slept all the way.

The exam was scheduled for 1:00 p.m., so Mom made us lunch before the exam. Letha was so weak that she could not lift the half-gallon milk carton to pour a glass of milk. I took her to the exam and sat in the car to read and wait for her to finish the exam so I would be available in case she could not finish and wanted to go home. Several people came out of the building, looking distressed. When Letha came out after a little over two hours, she told me that two of the five people had left the exam without completing it. One broke his pencils and threw them away as he left the exam. She said it was the strangest exam she had ever taken.

She was worn out, so we went straight home. When we walked into the house, my mom was on the phone. When she hung up, she said that it was Dr. Martzolf on the phone. He had just administered the exam and wanted to know if a girl named Foss was staying at our house. He had recognized the address on the exam registration papers. My parents had once lived next door to the Martzolfs, and they were good friends.

Dr. Martzolf had asked if Letha was well; she had looked ill to him. Mom had explained that she had mono. Dr. Martzolf said that he had called because she looked ill and he wanted her to feel better. He thought that knowing that she had just made the highest score on the Miller analogies test that he had seen in years of administering the exam would help.

That weekend, I told my mom that Letha and I wanted to get engaged. Mom was not enthusiastic about me being engaged to a sickly woman, but she got out two rings that she had been keeping for such an event. One was her engagement ring with a solitaire diamond. Dad had replaced it with a ring with a much larger oval-cut diamond on her twenty-fifth anniversary. The other was an old party ring that had a similar-sized central diamond with several smaller diamonds. The solitaire was an old-fashioned diamond, which was cut thicker than the modern style. The other ring had a modern-cut central diamond among the smaller diamonds. I picked the deeper cut because of the sentimental value. I took it to a jeweler to have it set in a new solitaire platinum ring.

Letha stayed in Normal for two weeks to recover from mono. Duncan Miller, the longtime high school band and chorus director, stopped by to see my mother about some school business. Mom introduced him to Letha. When he left, he said, "Happy to meet you, Mona" to Letha. He must have thought that her last name was "Nucleosis" and she was Greek. "Mona" became a nickname for Letha in our house for a while.

Dad had bought Bruce a new car when he graduated from college. Since they always treated us the same, they offered me my pick of any car in the low-priced three (Chevrolet, Pontiac, or Plymouth; Dad did not like Fords). When we went to the Pontiac showroom, there was a lemon yellow Catalina convertible in the showroom. I really liked the idea of a convertible. Dad was sure that it would flip over and kill me the first time I took it on the road. He kept saying, "You don't want the yellow one." I told him he was right, I wanted a "white" convertible. Mom sided with me.

They wanted to buy it early so they could take it to Mexico. At that time, Dad had a two-door Chevy sedan and Mom had a four-door Mercedes with four bucket seats. This trip was to be with Les and Wilma Cornick. Bruce was to be the driver and guide. The convertible had a split bench front seat and long doors, making it easier to get into the backseat than in Dad's Chevy. They were sure that they would have the top down most of the time in Mexico so they could get in and out easily. They wanted the car right away, prompting them to accept a Catalina with a Bonneville engine that was the only convertible available in the area. That was a lot of horsepower for a light car. It would fly away from stop signs.

When they got to Texas, they stopped in Amarillo for a six-pack of Pearl Beer. My grandfather had been on the board of directors of Pearl, and Mom still had Pearl stock. It was a family-held business. Dad claimed that they christened the car with Pearl when Les opened the beer because it sprayed onto the roof lining, making the car smell like beer for several days.

When they were in Mexico, the car hit a rock in the road that dented the transmission housing. There was a loud banging noise with every revolution of the drive shaft. They limped into Thomas and Charlie, the nearest town, at about five o'clock and found a garage. The mechanic at the garage discovered that the dented transmission housing was interfering with a bolt on the drive shaft. The housing would have to be removed, pounded back into the proper shape, and replaced.

The mechanic told his assistant, in Spanish, "If I fix this tonight, maybe the gringo will give me a big tip." Bruce had been speaking English until them. When he told the mechanic, in Spanish, that the "gringo" would give him a big tip, the mechanic was embarrassed into fixing it that night. This incident may be why the transmission went out three years later.

When I came back to Normal to take Letha back to school after she recovered, I learned that Bruce has just popped the question to Judy. Letha and I had set the date of June 24 for our wedding. We had told both sets of parents, and the date was spreading among the relatives.

Bruce had made arrangements to attend Middlebury College for summer school to prepare to go to the Middlebury campus in Madrid, Spain, to study for a master's degree in Spanish literature. He thought that June 24 was the perfect date for his wedding. After much discussion, he relented and chose June 17 for his wedding. It turned out to be a very busy month for all of us. Bruce was to be married in Normal, and I was to be married in Newcastle, Pennsylvania.

To make things more complicated, Letha's parents were evicted from the house they had rented for many years. It was being torn down to make room for a shopping center. They moved from Newcastle, Pennsylvania, to Boardman, Ohio, a suburb of Youngstown. Letha's mother worked at Lustig's, a very upscale shoe store in Youngstown. Letha's father was the regional salesman/distributor for Pillsbury for Northwest Pennsylvania and Northeast Ohio.

They moved into the new house three weeks before the wedding. The new house needed some painting and new curtains. Letha's parents were invited to Bruce's wedding so there was a lot to be done to the new house in a short time. I went to Ohio to help with the renovations. I was hanging curtain rods at three o'clock in the morning the night before we left to attend Bruce's wedding.

A week before Bruce's wedding, he came to Dad with severe abdominal pain and distention. The workup showed that he had a bowel obstruction. Dad called Dr. Ben Hoopes who did an exploratory laporotomy and discovered that a loop of small bowel had gotten caught under some adhesions from the prior colon surgery. Dr. Hoopes took down the adhesions to relieve the obstruction and the bowel was still viable, so he did not have to resect it. He sewed up the large abdominal incision, and Bruce was out of the hospital in two days.

Dr. Hoopes turned over the follow-up to Dad and told him to take out the sutures in about a week. Dad decided to leave the sutures in until after the honeymoon, one week after the wedding and two weeks after the surgery. He took out the sutures in Boardman, Ohio, the morning before Letha and I were married.

Bruce was married in the Baptist Church in Bloomington, where Judy was substitute organist. The wedding was followed by a reception in the basement of the church. The Baptists in Bloomington were strict prohibitionists so the reception was dry.

My parents threw another party at the house after the reception. They had ordered a generous supply of champagne for the party. Les Cornick took charge of the champagne. He brought the first bottle into the dining room to uncork it. The cork shot out of the bottle and hit the ceiling of the living room before striking the center of the five-foot-by-ten-foot double-pane picture window in the living room. Fortunately, it did not break the window.

Bruce and Judy left this reception for their honeymoon. The next day, I went with Letha and the Fosses back to Boardman to prepare for our wedding. The new curtains went up in the living and dining rooms. I did some touch-up painting of the woodwork on the first floor.

Letha's parents planned a dinner buffet at the house after the wedding for friends and family. My parents had me rent a party room at the motel, where they would be staying, for another champagne reception after the dry Presbyterian Church reception. The Presbyterians in Newcastle, Pennsylvania, were strict prohibitionists also.

Letha's family was divided when it came to alcohol consumption. Her father's relatives were strict Church of God and never touched a drop. Her mother's side were Presbyterians who looked for any reason to celebrate with a drink or two. There were several out-of-town guests from Normal, but a smaller crowd than the previous week. Because we thought that many of the guests were nondrinkers, Dad bought less champagne at the Ohio State Liquor store than he had the week before in Illinois.

After the wedding, Bruce retrieved my car from the hiding place behind the office of Letha's dentist. He put the top down before delivering it to the church. When we got in the car for him to drive us back to his car at the dentist's office, we stumbled into the backseat. The floor of the car was covered with empty Pearl beer cans. Les had saved them from the Mexico trip and had Bruce put them in the car. Fortunately, we did not kick any out of the car in front of the church as Les had hoped we would. By the time we pulled away from the church with the top down, the backseat of the car was full of rice. I think there was still rice in the car when I traded it in three years later.

After the church reception, everyone, except Letha and I, headed for the party at the motel in Boardman. Les took charge of the champagne again. His daughters Martha and Connie were there, and they worried that Les would drink too much so they kept emptying his glass into the potted flowers. He kept refilling it. When he opened the refrigerator door for more champagne, one bottle of champagne rolled out and smashed on the floor.

Everyone was surprised that the Foss side of the family found it appropriate to drink champagne at Letha's wedding even though they were teetotalers otherwise. The party soon ran short of champagne, so Dad sent Bruce to get more champagne. This was Bruce's first encounter with the Ohio State liquor stores. They could be very confusing when you wanted something specific, but he got more champagne. The reception lasted for almost two hours before most of the guests moved on to the Foss house.

The Fosses had a buffet dinner laid out. The house was small, but most of the guests sat around the living room and ate from their laps or stood in the kitchen holding their plates.

Years later, Letha's mom related a story from that evening. She was sitting next to Mrs. Wasson, Judy Wasson Barber's mother. Judy's mother leaned over to her and said something to the effect that both of the women were lucky that their daughters had snagged the Barber boys because their father was rich. Letha's mother was offended. She replied that her daughter was smart and attractive and could get anyone she wanted and that John was lucky to have convinced her to marry him.

The day after the wedding, Bruce and Judy headed east to Middlebury, Vermont, to prepare for his year of study in Madrid. The rest of the out-of-town guests headed back to Normal. Letha and I were already on our way to drive to California and fly to Hawaii, the wedding gift from my parents. I guess they felt generous because they had not had to pay for the two weddings.

Chapter 22

When Grandfather Bentzen died in St. Louis in 1960, Mom inherited his furniture. She had it all shipped to Normal and tucked most of it into our house. Every nook and cranny of the house was generously stuffed with furniture. During the spring of 1961, before the weddings, Bruce and I went through the house and divided Granddad's furniture.

When Letha and I returned from the honeymoon, we spent several days in Normal and then went to St. Louis to find an apartment. Mom came along to help find the apartment. My uncle Roy was working for a real estate company, so he insisted on showing us around town to help us find a place. Everything he showed us was too expensive for our budget. He was showing us what he would rent for himself, not student housing. We also learned that the apartment agents were adding a real estate agent commission to the rent on every apartment he showed us because he was there.

Roy had a cocktail party for us to introduce us to some of his friends. They had lots of suggestions for apartments—all were way above our budget. One friend suggested the building where they lived that was only a few blocks from the medical school. He told us that the owners were looking for some young tenants because the older tenants were wealthy and they all got drunk every night and abused the apartments. He thought that young people could not afford to drink that much so they would be better tenants.

Looking on our own, we found a two-bedroom upstairs flat in Richmond Heights, not too far from the medical school and the Washington U Hill Campus. It was $90 a month.

Mom took us downtown shopping, and we selected a bedroom suite. I had sold my sailboat in May to have the money to buy bedroom furniture. We went back to Normal to load up the hand-me-down furniture in a moving van. We returned to St. Louis ahead of the movers. Lambert's Furniture delivered the bedroom furniture to the apartment the day before the movers were scheduled to deliver so we could stay in the apartment before the other furniture came from Normal.

Once we were moved in, Mom and Dad came to visit. We heard, over and over, how plush we had it compared to when Dad was in medical school. My grandfather's furniture was mostly leather-topped mahogany tables and upholstered chairs. Letha called it early athletic club style.

We made the second bedroom into a study. I bought a flush door, an unfinished short cabinet, and two table legs to make a large desk. We used bricks and wood planks to make bookshelves on the back of the desk. A small table was used for the second desk. Letha and I traded desks, depending on what we were doing. Letha was a teaching assistant and graduate student in psychology at the Washington U Hill Campus.

I started medical school at the Barnes Hospital complex at the other end of Forrest Park from where we lived. Since Letha's classes were scattered throughout the day and my classes ran all day, she would drop me off at school and then go to the Hill Campus when she had classes. She would pick me up at five o'clock.

Letha had taken driver's training in high school and obtained a driver's license, but her father drove a company car that she was not allowed to drive. I had to teach her how to drive again. She practiced some in Normal and on our honeymoon. She loved the convertible with the big engine. It was a great advantage at the ubiquitous four-way stop signs in St. Louis.

Dad gave me his three-volume copy of the anatomy atlas by Spalteholz. This German atlas was supposed to have the best anatomy drawings ever done. He also gave me the skull that Uncle John Baber had acquired for him to use in medical school.

Dad was very busy with his practice at the height of his career. He was paying my tuition for medical school, which was $8,000 per year in the early sixties. Letha had a full tuition scholarship plus money for books because she was a teaching assistant. Eight of the eighty-six freshman medical students were married. Most of the other students lived in Olin dormitory next to the medical school or at the Phi Beta house three blocks away.

We lived on the trust fund that was set up for college that gave us about three thousand dollars a year. We managed to live comfortably while we were in school.

Chapter 23

When Dad was fifty-nine, he had a sudden gallstone attack. He went to Dr. Hoopes immediately and asked him to remove his gallbladder. Dr. Hoopes insisted on a full workup before he did the surgery. Dad told him that he had diagnosed many gallbladder attacks and knew one when he had it. He thought that further workup was foolish, but he went along with it anyway to please Dr. Hoopes.

Dad was in the hospital about five days after surgery and then went home to recuperate. Dr. Hoopes told him not to work until at least three weeks after surgery. Dad gave Cleta, his office nurse, three weeks of vacation and closed the office while he was to do nothing but loaf around the house.

Dad was listed in the telephone directory so his patients could call him with emergencies. With the office closed, they would call the house and demand to be seen. They offered to go to the office, the emergency room, or even come by the house. (At one time, there was a professor at ISNU named Brad Barber who had a PhD. He listed himself as Dr. Barber in the phone directory for one year, but got tired of being called at all hours of the day and night for medical care. Dad said it served him right for listing himself as a doctor. Dad made a clear distinction between MDs and PhDs.)

Dad refused to see patients because Dr. Hoopes had been adamant that he not practice for three weeks. Mom told the patients that Dr.

Dowd was covering his practice so they should call him. My mother got tired of arguing with them, so she packed some suitcases and drove them to the Ozarks in northern Arkansas. It was spring, and the redbuds and dogwood trees were in full bloom. She drove while they explored the area and fell in love with it as a retirement area. There was plenty of hunting and fishing and lots of places to explore.

Mom liked it so much that she found a house that was for sale that had a porch with a great view of Bull Shoals Lake so she bought it. She rationalized the purchase as a vacation house for the next five or six years until Dad retired.

Dad was working very hard because of the size of his practice. He was doing several surgical cases each week and running a full office every afternoon. After dinner, he made house calls until ten o'clock. His arthritic knees were bothering him, and his doctor had insisted that he cut back on sugar and salt.

He used Sucaryl in his coffee and iced tea. He insisted that this allowed him to spread a thick layer of jam or jelly on his breakfast toast for his sugar allowance. (His cousin in Richmond, whom we called "Uncle Worth," had taught Bruce and me to eat Aunt Clara's fresh homemade bread with a thick layer of butter that was hidden under a heavy layer of sugar. Dad's version of bread and jelly was much less caloric.)

Several of his friends and fellow doctors started telling him that he was working too hard and would soon work himself into the grave. My mother picked up on this and started working on him to retire. She convinced him that, if he wanted to retire to hunt and fish, he needed to do it when he was sixty.

There was a young doctor, Dr. Stutzman, who had started to practice in the little farm town of Carlock, Illinois, about ten miles from Normal. Dad sold him the office equipment and turned over the patient records and office lease in Normal. Dad abruptly retired, and they immediately moved to Bull Shoals, Arkansas, to make a clean break because of his experience after his gallbladder. They decided to keep the house in Normal for now with the idea that they might move back after his patients had become reconciled to his absence. They had planned the house for retirement.

Northern Arkansas was a very popular retirement area. There was an active newcomers group, and they made friends rapidly. They soon had a circle of friends that involved fourteen couples from all over the Midwest. They were people with the same values and political leanings. The men hunted and fished together. During the summer, they went together to pick wild fruit and berries. The women played bridge and had a book club. My mother promptly taught my father how to make jams and jellies so that she did not have to deal with the fruits and berries he picked. Dad was very proud of his jams and jellies and gave many of them away to friends and visitors.

The abrupt change from the everyday practice of medicine to retirement was hard for my father. He immediately hired a man to help him build a combination garage and workshop next to the house. When they leveled the ground to build the garage, the bottom of the shallow excavation was cooler than the surrounding ground. They killed three copperhead snakes in that depression in three days.

We came to visit at the time, and I decided to tear down an old low shed in the backyard that was used to store the lawn mower, gas cans, and snow tires. It would not be needed with the new garage. When I got down to the wooden pallets that made the floor of the shed, I flipped one over with a crowbar and found a coiled copperhead looking at me. I yelled to Dad about the snake. He approached the snake from behind with a spade and chopped off the head of the snake. After killing those four snakes, we did not see any for a long time.

Dad was restless for about a year after he retired. He was impatient with everything on TV except the news and sports. He would suddenly get up from his recliner and go out to the garage to tinker with things there. He spent a lot of time pounding nails into the wall to hang tools on. He organized and reorganized the tools on the walls. He had a Fiji Island coconut grater from his travels that he fitted onto a square wooden shaft so he could mount it in his vise to grate coconuts. There was always a good supply of grated coconut on hand.

On our trips to Florida, Dad learned shuffleboard, so he painted a court on our driveway in Normal. Once the garage in Arkansas was finished, he had the handyman build a shuffleboard court in the backyard. This involved a continuous pour of a concrete slab so that there would not be any joints or cracks to divert the disks. The slab was faced all around with a rock wall and had benches at both ends. Dad had lights installed to enable him to play at night.

Mom appealed to Bruce and me to come up with things for Dad to do, so I bought him a rock tumbler for Christmas. He used it once or twice and gave it up. He would load it with pebbles and grit and turn it on. After twenty-four hours, he would separate the pebbles and grit and change the grit size before running it another twenty-four hours. He was too impatient for this. Years later, when he was doing lapidary work in Arizona, he would tumble small rocks to make the end pieces for bolo ties or matching earrings for his stone pendants while he did the polishing of the larger rocks.

Bull Shoals Lake was built to supply energy for Arkansas, so the lake level was determined by rain along the White River and how much water was released to create hydroelectric power. This meant that the level of the water in the lake fluctuated. The boathouses on the lakeshore had to be moved up or down the bank every few days. Dad looked after the boathouse, mowed the grass, chopped firewood, and fished. Mom liked gathering with friends to play cards or have a drink while watching the sunset. Her idea of retirement was doing as little housework as possible and having lots of time for reading.

They had to go a mile into the village of Bull Shoals every day to get the mail at the post office, but the closest general grocery shopping was fifteen miles away in Mountain Home. Northern Arkansas was all dry, so everyone made an occasional whiskey run to the Missouri border, about twenty miles from Bull Shoals.

Bringing alcohol intro Arkansas was illegal. The sheriff would park near the state line where he could see anyone leaving the Borderline State Line Store and coming into Arkansas. He would stop cars and confiscate the liquor because it did not have Arkansas tax stamps. If you stopped at the liquor store at the state line, it was best to go on into Missouri for lunch and come back later. Alcohol with Arkansas state tax stamps was legal to purchase in Little Rock, but that was a four-hour drive on winding mountain roads.

Dad told me that with the right connections, you could buy moonshine throughout northern Arkansas. The revenuers were always raiding stills and busting up barrels of home brew, supposedly made for the legal purpose of "one's own consumption." It was hard to justify ten to twenty barrels for "one's own consumption." Dad always said that northern Arkansas would remain dry as long as the moonshiners could stagger out of the woods to vote it dry. They wanted to keep their business. Dad said that he never bought any because he was afraid that moonshine might have methanol in it. Methanol causes kidney damage, blindness, and death.

Dad bought a twenty-foot boat that had a straight-six Chevrolet engine with a J-prop drive. He could fish from it with a trolling motor or speed up the lake to visit other towns and local restaurants. The boat was very speedy and could easily tow two skiers. He bought two pairs of water skis for his frequent guests to use. He skied a few times when someone was there who could drive the boat, but soon gave it up. He would take people water-skiing if they knew how, but he was very impatient with anyone trying to learn.

The water that came out of the dam when electricity was being generated was from deep in the lake and always cold. The first ten miles of the White River below the dam was cold enough to support brown and rainbow trout and was kept stocked by the state. Dad loved to go downriver to rent a jon boat. He would anchor the boat across the current so two or three people could trail lines downstream. He covered the hook with canned corn for bait and trailed it downstream.

The river was low in the morning because very little power was generated late at night. When the power generation was turned on in the morning, the river started to rise. It took several hours for the rise to reach eight miles downstream. As the water rose, the anchor lines would tighten. Since the boat was anchored across the current, the upper side of the boat could swamp, dumping the occupants into the cold river. He always watched the riverbanks to be sure that we quit when the water started to rise.

Dad kept the trout he caught and learned how to smoke them. One of his friends in Bull Shoals was a butcher from Chicago, who had a special recipe for marinating fish. He confided the recipe to my father under strict secrecy. Les Cornick made him a smoker out of hot-air furnace ducts. He used a burner from a junked electric range. He wired the 220-volt burner to a 110-volt plug. The 110 current would make the burner hot enough to make wet sawdust smoke, but not flame. Les used shelves from old refrigerators for racks.

Dad would marinate the fish for ten to twelve hours and then smoke them for twenty-four hours. There were many sawmills in the area that were glad to give away a bucket of hardwood sawdust. Walnut, hickory, and maple were plentiful. Dad's smoked trout were great for an appetizer with a cocktail while watching the sunset over the lake from the front porch.

Their freezer was always stocked with a plentiful supply of smoked trout. When we visited, we always came home with frozen smoked trout wrapped in aluminum foil. We would have classmates in for a drink and pop a trout into the oven for ten to fifteen minutes to serve it to our guests.

Chapter 24

Mom and Dad moved to Arkansas in 1963. I was between my second and third year of medical school. Letha had finished two years of graduate school. She discovered a problem with her dissertation research because her adviser had recommended the wrong physiologic measurements. She had studied about thirty patients with recently diagnosed high blood pressure. This involved recording physiologic changes in pulse, blood pressure, galvanic skin response, etc.—in reaction to a loud noise. She had stacks of polygraph paper with the results, but she would have to repeat all of her research for her thesis because she discovered better ways to measure these responses.

She knew many of my classmates and considered herself an intellectual equal, or superior, to many of them. When she learned psychological testing, she had to take the tests first. Her IQ test was above the gradable level of the exam. She also recruited several of my classmates as test subjects for her practice testing, and she knew their results.

She was doing clinical psychology as part of her graduate school training and had become frustrated by the disdain shown to psychologists by psychiatrists. To maintain her interest in human behavior, she decided she wanted to be a psychiatrist, which meant that she had to go to medical school.

I went with her to see the director of admissions at the medical school. He was a retired general physician from Richmond, Missouri, who had his job because his son was an assistant dean. Letha explained why she wanted to go to medical school and told him that she had straight As in graduate school at Washington U. He told her that she did not need to go to medical school just because she was married to a medical student and that straight As in grad school did not indicate that she could do medical-school-level work. I put my hand on hers to keep her from leaping the desk and strangling him.

I learned from some of the faculty that the director of admissions was a figure and a paper shuffler who had no input in the selection of students. Letha applied and had the strong support of several of her professors.

We usually split holiday breaks between parents. This year, we went to Youngstown for Christmas with Letha's parents. On the way from Youngstown to Bull Shoals for New Year's Eve, we stopped in St. Louis to stay overnight. Letha's acceptance to medical school was in the mail.

We proceeded to Bull Shoals the next day and arrived at about ten o'clock on New Year's Eve. We watched TV with my parents until midnight. At midnight, I said that we had an announcement. I think my mother thought that Letha was pregnant, but Letha told them that she had been accepted to medical school. My father had drifted off to sleep again, so my mother woke him up to tell him. He said, "Good, is she qualified?" Letha showed him her letter, and he decided she must be qualified.

On New Year's Day, Dad and I went quail hunting. On the way, Dad said that he was glad that Letha would be in medicine. He went on to say that there were several fields that were suited for women, like pathology; ear, nose and throat; and dermatology. I warned him not to say that where she could hear it. I mentioned psychiatry, and he thought it would be OK. He told me again about his being offered a residency in psychiatry and a resulting promised position at Malcolm Bliss Hospital in St. Louis. He was not fond of psychiatry so he had turned it down. Letha had worked at Malcolm Bliss Hospital when she was a graduate student.

The next day, we got down to the nitty-gritty and asked if they would be willing to support both of us in medical school. My father was so glad to have two of us going into medicine that he agreed to continue to support us until Letha finished medical school. Letha started medical school as I started my fourth year. She was in the labs and classrooms. I was on the wards and clinics.

The next year, we were all in California for Christmas—Mom and Dad, Bruce and Judy, and Letha and me. There were no grandchildren yet.

Bruce and Judy had tried to have a child, but the years of Azulfidine medication for his ulcerative colitis had caused sterility. When they applied for permission to adopt, my brother was working at a think tank called Stanford Research Associates. His job required him to travel to foreign countries for months at a time to do evaluations, so the agencies decided that the home would not have two parents much of the time. Their application was turned down for that reason.

Bruce went to Iran for three months with Stanford Research Associates to advise the shah of Iran on ways improve agriculture to better feed the people of Iran. Bruce was "uniquely qualified" for the position, because he had worked one summer during high school as an agriculture worker for Funk's G-Hybrid Corn. He hoed weeds in hybrid corn patches that were isolated in bean fields where tractors could not go. They hand pollinated the corn using paper bags over the corn tassels and silks to produce hybrid corn. Strangely enough,

Stanford Research recommended growing corn in Iran to feed the people and the livestock. Opium poppies were not good for either one although they brought more income to the farmers.

He went with a group to Argentina to do a study about transportation into the interior. The government asked for advice on whether it would be better to build roads through the jungles or develop better airports in the interior. I do not remember what they recommended or whether the government followed their advice.

Judy was enrolled in Stanford University when Bruce had this job. She decided to drop out of her freshman year to go with Bruce on one of these trips. When she returned, she was allowed to restart her college work at Stanford. Several months later, she dropped out again to join Bruce on another trip. When she asked to be readmitted this time, her request was denied because she had dropped out twice.

Judy went on to earn a degree in computers from De Anza College and then got her master's degree in theater from San Jose State. She got a job doing secretarial and administrative work on computers at Stanford. She had taken courses in Word and Excel at De Anza. She also served as a docent at the Stanford Museum, becoming an expert on the Rodin sculptures there.

Judy had just finished her master's thesis on the use of art in theater sets. In the process of doing her thesis research, she had decided to become an opera singer. This would require her going back to school to major in music. She would also need to have a regular voice teacher, which was expensive. She was about twenty-five years old and had not had any formal voice training.

My mother thought that an opera singer had to have years of voice training before they were twenty. Mom was dead set against it and refused to support her through the training. This caused immediate friction between Letha and Judy because Judy knew that my parents were supporting Letha in medical school. This remained a source of friction for years to come.

My father tried to keep out of this argument, but silently backed my mother. He later told me that he thought it was a bad idea and that Judy needed to take care of Bruce rather than pursue a career. It was the one time that they did not treat us exactly alike. I think that if Judy had made some other career choice, they might have backed her. I think that Judy's history at Stanford played a role in my parents' decision not to back Judy for her singing career.

In the fall of my third year of medical school, my mother called me early in the morning before I left for school. She told me that she was bringing my father to St. Louis to see Dr. McCarroll for his back. Dr. McCarroll was the classmate of my father's who had gone into orthopedics and was a professor at Washington U.

Dad had been going to a chiropractor in Mountain Home, Arkansas, for pain in his lower back. It was so bad he could hardly get out of bed or stand up straight. After the chiropractor worked on him, he could stand up straight and walk without pain. The next day, he had bad pain again and returned to the chiropractor who got him walking again.

The morning my mom called, the pain had returned and Dad decided to see an orthopedist. He had seen Dr. McCarroll again at his last medical class reunion and decided to consult him. Dr. McCarroll diagnosed a ruptured lumbar disc and put him in the hospital for spinal traction to see if they could avoid surgery.

Dr. McCarroll was president of the American Orthopedic Society that year, so he had to leave town to run the national meeting of the Society. He told my father that his residents would watch over him. If the pain did not improve, he would return from the meeting to do surgery to remove his herniated lumbar disk.

The pain did not abate except briefly, immediately after the traction treatments. The residents made rounds every afternoon right after his traction treatment, so he was feeling somewhat better. His pain was bad enough that he could not sleep at night until about 5:00 a.m. The residents made rounds at about six o'clock and found him sleeping so they did not awaken him. They reported to Dr. McCarroll that he was doing better.

Saturday afternoon, when Dr. McCarroll returned from his meeting, he came to see Dad. Dad told him that he was no better than before and that the pain was wearing him down. Dr. McCarroll called the OR and scheduled him for emergency surgery to remove his disk.

That night, Dad could not urinate and became distended. This was not uncommon for older men after surgery. The anesthesiologists usually gave the patients atropine to dry up pulmonary secretions to prevent pneumonia after anesthesia. A side effect of the atropine made it impossible for the patient to urinate until it wore off. They had to catheterize him.

When Dr. Justin Cardonnier, the chief of urology, examined Dad, he found a large prostate, and they decided to do a transurethral resection (TUR) to treat this short-term obstruction in the postoperative period and hopefully avoid future problems. They did not find any evidence of cancer in the resected tissues, which meant that he only had benign prostatic hypertrophy.

That was the beginning of his long battle with prostate problems. The prostate continued to grow, so Dad had to have a TUR about every five years. He did well for a while after surgery, but would eventually have trouble. When he had to catheterize himself to relieve obstruction, it was time for another TUR.

My parents kept the house in Normal for several years, thinking that they would live there in the summers. They had many friends in Bloomington–Normal and wanted to keep in touch with them. Maintaining the house in Normal while they were in Arkansas became difficult, so they put the house on the market.

When it was built in 1947–48, it was one of the most expensive houses in Normal. There were many new construction techniques, and the cost of postwar materials made it unique and expensive.

There was an aggressive real estate broker in Bloomington who helped convince them to sell the house, so they listed it with her. At that time, in the early 1960s, there was not much movement in real estate in Normal in the upper price range. No new doctors or lawyers were coming to town, and the university faculty could not afford it.

There was a retired nurse in Bloomington who had worked for many years with my father at Brokaw Hospital and had been in the delivery room when I was born. When she retired from hospital nursing, she took a job in private nursing, caring for a very wealthy widower. This man owned a manufacturing company and had invested in several large farms near Bloomington. This nurse took very good care of him and would drive him to his farms to check with his tenant farmers. She saw to his needs while his family largely ignored him. When he died, he left his millions to the nurse.

By the time she wanted the house, she had developed diabetes and was overweight. The combination caused her to spend most of her time in a wheelchair. She wanted a house that was on one floor so she could get around in her wheelchair.

She liked the house, but would not deal through their real estate agent. The agent was the daughter-in-law of the man whom she had looked after. The agent and her husband had sued her to break the will, claiming that the nurse had fooled a senile old man into changing his will and that the old man had not been competent at the time the will was changed.

My father happened to be the old man's doctor and had seen him regularly during the time in question. He was called as expert witness for the trial and told me later that he had used his knowledge of Latin to testify that the old man was "compos mentis" at the time the will was rewritten.

When the problem surfaced that the buyer would not deal with the agent, the agent made it known that she did not want to deal with the buyer either. The agent dropped out and allowed the sale to take place. Such is life in a small town.

After the nurse moved in, she decided to put an intercom system in the house so she would not have to go in her wheelchair to answer the door. She could talk with the caller at the door from anywhere in the house. We learned that it took workers about three months with jackhammers and concrete chisels to wire the house for the intercom. She could easily afford the work, but it was an inconvenience.

For the next several years, Mother and Dad rented an apartment in a new building that had just been built on the old country club grounds at the edge of town. They would go to Normal during the holiday season and give parties for their friends. The family would gather at the apartment for Christmas.

During my internship at St. Luke's Presbyterian Hospital in St. Louis, Dad decided that I should learn to fly an airplane so that we could visit them more often in Bull Shoals. There as a small gravel airstrip near Flippin, Arkansas, that was only a few miles from Bull Shoals. (It was also near the Whitewater Estates that were later made famous by President Clinton and Hillary.)

I mentioned becoming a pilot to Dr. Meader and Dr. McGinnis who were both surgeons at St. Luke's and pilots. They told me that although they were pilots, they thought that doctors had a very poor track record as pilots. Doctors were the leading profession among pilots who were killed in private plane crashes. The reason was that some doctors did not take time to properly maintain their airplanes and tended to fly in bad weather because of busy schedules. They advised against becoming a pilot. Letha was not very happy with the idea of my piloting planes either.

Several times, while I was at the FDA and during my residency, Dad gave me the money to fly us commercially to Little Rock. He sent a one-engine plane from Flippin to pick us up and bring us to Bull Shoals. My experiences in that single-engine plane flying over the Ozarks did not encourage me to take up flying.

Chapter 25

After my internship, I enlisted in the public health service and was assigned to the Food and Drug Administration in Washington, DC. Mom and Dad came to visit us for the holidays during our first year in Washington. Letha had transferred from Washington University in St. Louis to George Washington University in DC for her clinical years.

Dad learned that Dr. Brian B. Blades was chief of surgery at GW. He had known him as a fellow student at Washington University Medical School, so he decided to pay him a call. Dr. Blades had gained fame as a preeminent cardiothoracic surgeon and by operating on President Eisenhower while he was in office.

Dad went to the GW hospital and found Dr. Blades's office. He introduced himself to Dr. Blades's secretary and was told he would have to make an appointment to see Dr. Blades, because Dr. Blades was very busy. My dad told her that he was an old friend of Dr. Blades and just wanted to say hello to "Blackie".

When Dad called him "Blackie" the secretary told him that he must be a long time friend of Dr. Blades because no one called him "Blackie" anymore. Dr. Blades had gotten the nickname "Blackie" in medical school because of his wavy black hair. What little hair Dr. Blades had now was white. She called into his office and Dr. Blades had her show Dad right in.

They talked for some time, and Dad told Dr. Blades that his daughter-in-law was a junior student at GW. Dr. Blades told Dad that he would look out for her. Several months later, while Letha was on the surgery rotation, she was assigned to scrub with Dr. Blades in surgery. It was customary for the students and house staff to introduce themselves to the surgeon at the start of surgery.

When Dr. Blades heard Letha's last name, he asked if she was Harry Barber's daughter-in-law. When she said yes, he had the resident move down the table and had Letha stand opposite to him. He spent the entire case explaining what he was doing, step by step, to Letha. This did not go over well with the other students and house staff, but I am sure that Dr. Blades meant well for Letha. She graduated with honors, Alpha Omega Alpha, the national medical honorary, and was a member of Smith, Reed, Russell, the local medical honorary.

While I was working for the FDA in Washington, Mom decided that we should all go to the Virgin Islands for the Christmas holidays. Mom and Dad, Bruce and Judy, and Letha and I all met in Miami and flew to St. Thomas. We spent several days there before flying to St. Croix for a week in an old plantation house on the west end of the island. Mom had booked it through AAA who advertised it as gracious life in a gloriously restored plantation house on the beach.

We arrived on the day specified on our itinerary, but the plantation was not expecting us. The fancy rooms in the house were full. They put us in rooms behind the house that had been remodeled from concrete block slave quarters by adding primitive bathrooms to the back side of the building. The bathrooms had bare concrete floors, and the commodes were recessed into the floor so low that it was like squatting on the floor.

Dinners were in the main house, but the food was rationed. One day, we saw the owner spear fishing on the beach. He had speared two large Caribbean lobsters. That night, the dinner was surf OR turf. The lobsters were divided into slices about an inch and a half thick, and the steaks were fillet sized. When the hostess brought the food to the table, we were told that we could have one slice of lobster OR one steak. The vegetable for dinner was tree squash, picked from the tree behind the house. We discovered that the family was trying to live all year from the profits of a three-month tourist season.

Dad was very unhappy with this place and blamed it on Mom's favorite travel agent at AAA in St. Louis. He did enjoy swimming in the crystal-clear waters of the beach. With diving masks, we could see the anchor ropes of the boats anchored fifty yards from the beach.

There was an honor bar with a notebook to record the drinks you made for yourself. When the supply of limes for daiquiris ran out, they would send one of the black servant boys to the lime tree for more.

Letha had a sore throat and a cough, but we did not have any cough medicine and we were miles from town with no transportation. Since the cough syrup, elixir of terpin hydrate, tastes just like Grand Marnier, she decided to see if the latter would calm her cough. She drank a shot of it just before going back to the room at night, and it did help her sore throat.

Judy saw the drink recorded in the drink book the next morning and immediately told Dad that she thought Letha was becoming an alcoholic because she was sneaking drinks before bedtime. Dad confronted Letha about it and learned the reasoning behind the Grand Marnier and was glad to know that it helped her cough.

Letha and Judy never got along well, and things like this made it worse. Judy was condescending to Letha, talked down to her, and was very passive aggressive toward her. Letha would be nice and try not to notice it, but after so much, she would lash out at Judy with some decimating remark that put Judy in her place, at which time Judy would deny the passive-aggressive digs she had been making and blame Letha for an unprovoked attack. Judy loved to play this game.

The next year, Mom decided she wanted to see Central America. Letha was three months pregnant in February that year, but wanted to make the trip. Bruce and Judy were living in Belgium where Bruce was working for Dole Pineapple Company. We flew to Miami and met Mom and Dad for the flight to San Juan, Costa Rica. We got our rental car and stayed in a motel on the edge of town. The first day there, we drove up Mount Iratzu, a high volcanic peak. Since his first trip to Hawaii, Dad was fascinated by volcanoes. We walked down into the caldera of the volcano and peered into the steaming lava pit. Everything, especially our shoes and pants cuffs, was covered in gray ash from a recent eruption. The trees were all covered with ash, and everything was a monotone gray.

On the way down the mountain, we were stopped by a group of boys selling green and white striped melons. Dad wanted a watermelon, so he asked the lead boy if they were *sandia* (Spanish for watermelon) and the boys said "Si!" He bought one for about a dollar, and we proceeded to look for a restaurant.

We found a good-looking restaurant and went in. The menu was in Spanish. Bruce was the Spanish linguist of the family, but they had not yet arrived. Dad spotted a word that he recognized, *tortilla*, and ordered it. The waiter asked him how many he wanted, and he said "Uno." The rest of us ordered the soup of the day, mondongo soup. It turned out to be a vegetable soup with tripe in it—not the best thing to eat in a foreign country. They brought out one tortilla for Dad. He remembered the word for "five," *cinco*, and ordered five more.

They had *helado* (ice cream) for dessert, so we all ordered it. Dad asked if it was chocolate ice cream by asking, "Con chocolate?" The waiter said "si" and gestured whether everyone wanted "con chocolate?" We all said "si." Some of us had been drinking coffee, but they immediately gathered up the coffee cups and put out new cups. We saw it coming but could not stop it. They served us strawberry ice cream along with hot chocolate to drink.

Bruce and Judy arrived that evening, and we picked them up at the airport. We had put the watermelon in the refrigerator at the motel and expected to eat it with Bruce and Judy that night. The motel kitchen had a big knife that was just right to cut the watermelon. When I cut into the melon, it was white inside. It was a giant squash. Bruce said we had been bilked because none of us knew Spanish. I told him that the kids had said it was *sandia*, which was one word that we all knew.

It was close to Dad's birthday, so we went to the grand hotel in downtown San Jose for a fancy dinner. When it was time for dessert, Dad saw cherries jubilee on the menu and ordered it. It was near Washington's birthday, so we all ordered cherries jubilee. The chef came to our table and apologized that they were out of cherries. He offered to make it with some fresh strawberries instead. Dad was a big fan of strawberries, so he agreed to have strawberries jubilee. When they served it, the strawberries had cooked into a hot strawberry jam that was served over the ice cream—good but not quite the same.

After several days in Costa Rica, we flew to Guatemala City. Our tour of the capital was abbreviated because of a civil war. We were awakened on our first night by a running gun battle that went down the street in front of the hotel. The army was chasing a man down the esplanade in the middle of the street. We watched from our hotel window as they worked their way up the street about a block apart with the escaping man running from tree to tree and occasionally shooting at the following soldiers. The soldiers would fire back as the chase went on down the street. No one appeared to be a good shot.

The next day, we were told that we could not visit the museum because the war was in that part of town that day. We did tour the capitol building where we were accompanied by an armed uniformed guard who appeared to be about fifteen years old. He was carrying a rifle over his shoulder, but played with a yoyo most of the time he was with us.

We went to Antigua and then to Panajachel on Lake Atitlan before spending three days in Chichicastenango (city of the castor beans). Dad used about five rolls of film in Chichi. Most of the people were dressed in colorful native garb and doing activities out of the past. The men planted corn by hand, putting a primitive hoe in the ground to open a hole into which they placed three kernels of corn, saying one for the birds, one for the gods, and one for the corn. The women wove colorful fabrics on back looms suspended from trees or posts. Dad enjoyed taking pictures of the live chickens and unusual vegetables on market day.

There were many children running everywhere, but the babies never cried. Dad determined that it was because the mothers carried the babies everywhere in a sling on their backs. When it was feeding time, they just swung the sling around to feed the baby.

We were there during Lent so all the outlying villages had processions to bring the saint from their local church to Chichi to be blessed by the priests. These processions had bands composed of primitive marimbas, reed flutes, skin and pottery drums, and sometimes brass horns. The shaman would lead the procession and dance around the statue of the saint on the steps of the church, carrying incense and exploding fireworks. After the priests blessed the saint, the shaman would take a collection from the crowd that had gathered. Dad noticed that the priests all contributed to the collection.

Dad led a visit to the Methodist hospital. When we noticed that there were no patients in the hospital, the director said that they had all left to go to the market. There was not a slipper or a toothbrush left behind to suggest that there were any patients to come back.

On the way back through town, we passed the Catholic hospital where there was a line of people sitting on their suitcases, waiting to get into the hospital. We learned that the Methodist hospital required their patients to denounce their pagan religion and declare themselves Christian before they could enter the hospital. The Catholics took in the pagans and taught them Christianity while they were in the hospital.

My father thought it was wrong to hold medical care hostage to religious belief but did not go back to the Methodist hospital to tell them. Dad had a strong moral commitment to care for anyone in need, regardless of race or religion, including prisoners and enemy combatants.

From Guatemala we flew to Merida, Mexico. This trip included several airlines that we had never heard of, like Sasha and Taca. We rented a car and drove to the Mayan ruins at Uxmal and Kabah near Merida. Letha had trouble climbing the pyramids because her pregnancy aggravated her congenital heart defect. Some older ladies chided her for not being able to climb up a stairway inside one of the pyramids fast enough for them. Dad was fascinated by the building skills of the Mayan people and the extent of the ruins so he took several rolls of photos.

We drove to Chichen Itza to see more pyramids and the giant cenote. This large deep pond was where drugged twelve-year-old virgins, born during the short month of the Mayan calendar, were drugged and sacrificed by jumping to their deaths wearing enough gold ornamentation to sink them so they did not swim or float back up. They were to become brides of the gods. Disappearing and not resurfacing proved their acceptance by the gods. Many of the gold adornments have been excavated and taken to the Peabody Museum in Boston. Dad was fascinated by the history and the barbarism of beheading the losing ball team after the championship game in their mixture of soccer and basketball.

We stayed in a hacienda run by a domineering woman who also controlled the taxicabs and the airport. The Mexicans followed their custom of taking a siesta after lunch, so tourists were expected to nap after lunch. This was fine since it was so hot, but there was a macaw in a cage in the courtyard of the hacienda that shrieked every few minutes from two o'clock until four o'clock, making a siesta impossible.

From Chichen Itza we flew to Cancun on a DC-3. The airport was a limestone gravel strip with a large wind sock to tell the pilot the direction and strength of the wind. The woman at the hotel loaded everyone into taxis to the air terminal that consisted of a twenty-by-thirty-foot open-air thatched roof over two-foot-high walls. There was an entry gap in the wall on one side and a "boarding gate" exit gap on the tarmac side. The woman collected all the tickets and told us to wait.

The plane made a pass to check the wind sock, landed upwind, and taxied to about one hundred feet from the thatched roof before shutting off the port engine. The door stairway was lowered, and about twenty passengers deplaned. Their luggage was unloaded and brought to a spot near the thatched roof.

There were no seat assignments, so people started walking toward the plane to get good seats. Suddenly there was a woman's voice from a loud megaphone saying, "Has your flight been called? Go back to the gate area until your flight is called!"

Cancun had been hit by a hurricane the summer before and had only partially recovered. Only three of the hotels were open. The only restaurants were the hotel dining rooms. Our dining room had five choices of meat or fish with pico de gallo sauce and the same five choices with a kind of chocolate "molé" sauce.

By this point on the trip, I had developed a bad case of "tourista." On Dad's recommendation, I was consuming large quantities of Pepto-Bismol. I was the only one of our group with this problem. Someone in Cancun told Dad that a common cause of "tourista" in Mexico was eating too much papaya. I love papaya and had been eating half of a large Mexican papaya for breakfast every day. Once I stopped eating it, my gastrointestinal problems improved. Dad had never seen a case of papaya gastroenteritis. Apparently, there are large quantities of the enzyme papain in papaya; too much papaya eats the lining of the gastrointestinal tract.

We all flew from Merida to Miami and went our separate ways. Bruce had a connection to Brussels, so he checked his luggage through and did not have to go through customs. The rest of us went to baggage claim to go through customs. As we claimed our bags, I spotted Bruce's suitcase on the carousel. I told the baggage handlers that it was supposed to be on a plane to Belgium. The tag indicated the flight number, but it had already left the gate. The bag finally caught up with him in Belgium several days later.

Chapter 26

When Dad retired and moved to Bull Shoals, Arkansas, he began looking for hobbies to keep him busy. He liked photography, but soon exhausted his supply of things in Arkansas that he was interested in photographing. Polishing stones was too boring.

He had a new friend who was a ham radio operator. Dad decided to become a ham operator so his friend started teaching him about ham radio. He spent hours studying the electronics of transmitters and receivers and bought a machine to help him learn the international Morse code.

This code machine played perforated paper tapes that created coded messages. A dial on the console could change the speed of the tapes, and there were also practice tapes for sending code by repeating the codes with a key. Dad eventually reached the required eighteen or twenty words per minute to pass his test. He became a novice ham operator. After a year, he passed another test to become a full-fledged ham operator. He enjoyed talking with English-speaking people from all over the world, and it kept him busy during the evening hours.

After a while, he decided that I should become a ham so that we could converse by radio. He gave me a Heathkit multiband radio transceiver kit along with the power supply kit for me to assemble. He included both real and dummy antennas.

I was working at the FDA in Washington at the time while Letha was doing her last two years of medical school at George Washington University. We lived next door to the FDA in a high-rise apartment. Letha was busy every night studying so I had lots of time to build the radio and power supply. Dad sent me his code machine to use to learn to send and receive code at twenty words per minute.

As soon as I completed assembling the radio, I plugged it in and turned it on. There was a sparking sound, and smoke came out of the back of the radio. I shut it down and opened the back. There was a brown spot on one of the circuit boards, and a few resistors and capacitors were partially melted. I checked the board and found that one of the wires was too long so that it was touching the circuit board in the wrong place. It had shorted out part of the circuit.

I consulted the directions to see what parts I needed and went to Radio Shack to get new ones. Once the bad parts had been replaced and checked for loose wires, I tried the transceiver again and it worked. I was able to listen to ham operators in code and voice, but I could not legally transmit. I had a twelve-foot-long "Texas Bug Catcher" antenna that was meant to be mounted on the rear bumper of a car. I laid it horizontally on wooden blocks on our balcony where it was not visible from the outside. The antenna had a large coil that could be tuned to make the antenna usable for various transmission wavelengths. I practiced the code with Dad's machine and also on the radio tuned to a frequency that broadcasted practice code. I did not get up to qualifying speed before it was time for Letha to graduate from medical school and for us to move to Richmond, Virginia, for me to start my residency.

Once my residency started, I was using all of my time to study ophthalmology and get used to living in our own house. Letha was pregnant when she graduated in June. Scott was born on the eighteenth of August so I was very busy. I stopped practicing code and soon lost what proficiency I had obtained and did not have time to listen to other hams. Dad was disappointed, but knew that I had to study a lot for my residency. By the time I had finished my residency and fellowship and had time to practice code, Dad had given up the ham radio.

Chapter 27

Dad always asked me about what I was learning in medical school. When I was on the obstetrics rotation, learning to deliver babies, he asked me if they still had a basin of cold water in the room during deliveries. I told him that there were three basins—one with soapy water, one with cold sterile water, and one that was empty. He asked me what the cold sterile water was for. I told him that they had never explained to us why it was there.

He told me that he had always wondered about it himself until he delivered a baby one day that he could not get to take a first breath. He had used the oral bulb syringe to suck out the mouth to clear any secretions blocking the airway, he had hung it upside down by the ankles and swatted it on buttocks and the soles of the feet, and he had run his knuckles up and down the baby's spine to stimulate it. It would not breathe, so he plopped the baby's bottom into the cold water. It took a deep breath and kept on breathing.

Scott was born in the second month of my residency in Richmond, Virginia. Letha had changed obstetricians when we moved to Richmond in July so we did not have much rapport with the new doctor. I insisted on being in the delivery room because Letha wanted me there. Laypeople could be excluded from the delivery room, but since she and I were both doctors, it was permitted so he reluctantly agreed.

The anesthesiologist who was attending to Letha noticed signs of fetal distress and insisted that the obstetrician hurry the delivery. The obstetrician said that the labor had stalled because the head was in the wrong position. He would have to rotate the baby with forceps to get the head in the right position. The back of the head has to be up—he thought it was down. He rotated the head and proceeded to deliver the baby with the forceps. He discovered that he had misread the feel of the skull bones and the head was now wrong so he had to rotate it more to get it in the "occiput up" position. By the time the head was out, he discovered that the umbilical cord was wrapped around the neck three times (the third time from the rotations.) He cut the cord early and delivered a very blue baby boy.

In the process of the high forceps delivery, the doctor had created a large (third degree) vaginal laceration that was profusely bleeding. The doctor handed the baby to me to revive so that he could concentrate on stopping Letha's bleeding. I was glad that I had scrubbed in and glad that I had delivered about thirty babies during my internship.

I held the baby upside down and used the oral syringe to suck out his mouth and throat. I swatted him on the butt and on the bottoms of his feet as was usually done to make a baby breathe and cry. He would not breathe. I rubbed my knuckles up and down his spine like I had been taught. Still nothing. Finally, I remembered what my father had told me about the basin of cold water. I dropped the baby's bottom into the cold water, and he gasped a deep breath. He continued to breathe and immediately started to go from blue to purple to pink. I found a pulse that was strong and steady. Dad had saved his only grandchild by telling me about the basin of cold water.

We named him Scott after his uncle in Pennsylvania.

We had no way to tell whether Scott suffered brain damage from oxygen deprivation because of the cord around the neck three times. Letha's studies in psychology had taught her a lot about brain damage. She was worried that Scott's IQ would be low and that his muscular coordination would be poor. He might have cerebral palsy.

When his IQ was finally tested in high school, it was about 145. Scott was slow to walk, but his coordination became good enough that he was able to play zone conference tennis tournaments in grade school.

I got to teach Dad a few things about modern medicine. One time when I was visiting in Arkansas while I was an intern and could write prescriptions, he asked me to give him a prescription for chloramphenicol to take when he got a cold. I told him that "chloro" did not work for cold viruses. He answered back that it worked for "large viruses."

I explained that what he knew as large viruses were now called Chlamydia and that colds were caused by small viruses. Besides, chloramphenicol was known to cause aplastic anemia as a rare side effect that was usually fatal. No one was prescribing "chloro" anymore except in life-and-death cases. He told me that he had read about the aplastic anemia and thought it was some professor's excuse to write a paper at the "ivory tower." I told him that I had seen several cases of aplastic anemia that were thought to be from chloramphenicol. I did not write him the prescription.

Dad was a lifelong smoker. During his years in the Arctic, he smoked a pipe and brought back several pipes on which he had carved faces on the outside of the bowl. While working in the office, he would take one or two drags on a cigarette between patients as he passed through the laboratory between his two examining rooms. Each cigarette was good for four to six drags because it burned while he was seeing patients. He would average a little over a half pack per afternoon that he actually smoked. He also smoked between surgical cases and between house calls when he was driving.

He tried several times to quit, but those times only lasted a few days. After his bypass surgery in 1973, he quit for almost a year on orders from Dr. Cooley. Then he decided that he was living on borrowed time because he would have been dead without the bypass surgery. He decided that he might as well enjoy his extra final years by smoking. After he retired, Mom would not allow him to smoke in the house. He rolled down the window in his car when he smoked, but the car still smelled of smoke.

He did not believe the connection between smoking and cancer, even lung cancer. When I challenged him about this, he told me that he had a long-term patient who never smoked a cigarette in her life who died of lung cancer. She probably had a cylindroma of the lung, which is a rare form of cancer of the bronchioles in the lung that is not related to smoking. He still clung to this excuse for continuing to smoke. (Adenocarcinoma of the lung is the type that has been linked to smoking, as are cancer of the tongue and bladder.)

Chapter 28

As the family scattered, Bruce and Judy to California and Letha and I to Washington, the apartment in Normal lost its usefulness so they let it go. They spent all year in Bull Shoals, Arkansas. There were three houses on their "street," and they spent a lot of time with both of their neighbors until the next-door neighbor became paranoid and began accusing both of his neighbors of stealing his tools and lying to him.

Dad's knees were starting to bother him when he walked. Dr. McCarroll ordered X-rays and discovered that his knee cartilages were thin and densely calcified. The doctor told Dad to give up hunting because if he fell while he was hunting and tore or cracked one of these cartilages, he might not be able to walk out of the woods. He had given up golf at about the time he retired because the arthritis in his hands made him afraid that the club would slip out of his hands and might injure someone. Dad continued to fish, maintain the boat, move the boathouse, mow the lawn, chop wood, and otherwise remain very active; but he quit berry picking and hunting in the woods.

One Christmas, Mom and Dad were visiting us in Richmond, Virginia. I was on call for the middle days of the holiday break. Dr. Kemper Humphries, one of the other third-year residents, called me the day before Christmas. He was seeing a woman in the emergency room who had punctured her cornea with a nail while putting up

Christmas decorations. She was now developing a cataract. This traumatic cataract could swell within twenty-four to forty-eight hours to a size that would block the outflow of fluid from the eye and cause acute glaucoma. Kemper had advised her to have the cataract removed immediately to avoid this problem.

She was a single parent with two small children at home. She had been decorating for her children's Christmas and would not spoil their Christmas by being in the hospital, but she agreed to come in the day after Christmas for surgery. Her mother would watch the children. I would be on call starting Christmas Day while Kemper planned to be at his parents' house in Charlottesville.

I called the operating room and scheduled surgery for 9:00 a.m. on December 26 and then called an attending surgeon to assist me at surgery. The doctor I called told me that since I had done this procedure before, I should go ahead and aspirate the cataract and call him if there was any difficulty. I asked my dad if he wanted to come with me to watch a cataract extraction. He could watch with his one eye through the monocular observer arm of the microscope. He was looking for something to do, so he jumped at the opportunity.

We met the woman in the emergency room and walked her through the admitting process before taking her directly to the operating room. Mrs. Keagle, the operating room nurse for ophthalmology, was there and had everything ready. I introduced my father and explained that he was a physician so it was all right for him to be in the operating room. I told her who the attending surgeon was and what he had told me about calling him. This was not uncommon in 1970.

The patient was prepped and draped, and I made a retrobulbar (behind the eye) injection to numb the area and keep the eye from moving during surgery. A needle was placed into the eye, between the iris and the cornea, and attached to a bag of saline to maintain a constant pressure in the eye to keep the eye inflated to its normal shape.

I made a small incision at the edge of the cornea at twelve o'clock (closest to me at the head of the table). I used a sharp needle through this incision to cut an X in the front of the lens capsule to open the lens. Then I placed a small hollow blunt needle on a syringe, through the incision into the center of the lens. The lens had become swollen and cloudy from the injury, and the lens tissue was the consistency of Jell-O.

I gently aspirated the contents of the lens into the syringe until the capsule was empty and the red reflection through the pupil opening was completely clear. Only the clear capsule of the lens remained. I pulled the needles from the eye and examined the incision. It was water tight, but I found that it leaked if I put pressure on the back edge of the incision. I put in one tiny stitch of 10-O nylon to make the incision water tight. The needle tract for the irrigation needle did not leak, so no stitch was needed there. The entire procedure had taken less than fifteen minutes.

On the way home, Dad told me that he had never seen eye surgery before and he thought that what I had just done was the slickest, most delicate surgery he had ever seen. He now understood why I had chosen ophthalmology over general surgery. He had been very disappointed when I made the choice because it meant that I would not be coming home to follow in his footsteps.

That was at the time when I was deciding whether I would do a fellowship after my residency. If I wanted to teach in academic medicine, I needed to do a fellowship in one of the specialties of ophthalmology. I had interviewed for fellowships in San Francisco and Boston, and I was also applying in Miami. I decided to bring this up at dinner that night to feel out my parents about being partially on their support for two more years of study.

Dad's immediate reaction was that I had been at the FDA for two years and in my internship and residency for four more years after I graduated from medical school. It was time to go treat some people. He said, "Enough studying. Go treat some people!"

I told him that I had been accepted for the fellowship at Massachusetts Eye and Ear Infirmary in Boston and that Mass Eye and Ear was part of the Massachusetts General Hospital and Harvard Medical School.

This rang a bell with Dad because he still read the *New England Journal of Medicine*. Every week, there was a report of a clinical pathological conference from Mass General. Dad knew that Mass General was one of the best hospitals in the country.

He asked me, in a tone of disbelief, if I could really go there. I told him that I had been accepted and that two years of Harvard on my curriculum vitae would do a lot for a career in academic medicine. He decided that training at Harvard would be OK.

Chapter 29

Near the end of my fellowship in Boston, I accepted a faculty position at the University of Texas in Galveston. Letha, Scott, and I went to Galveston to look for a house. Mom and Dad drove to Galveston to babysit and help us decide on a house. We stayed in the Flagship Hotel. This hotel had been built on the remains of an amusement park pier, extending from the seawall out over the Gulf of Mexico at Twenty-Fifth Street. The amusement park had been destroyed by Hurricane Carla.

Dad always looked for someone to talk with. When he talked with the hotel manager, he learned that the hotel was built in an unusual way. Each floor was completed and then jacked up for another floor to be built beneath it. Eventually, it was about seven stories high. The balconies on the northeast side were directly over the water and had signs on the railings saying that fishing from the balconies was prohibited. When we stayed there, there were many fishing lines hanging from these balconies. (Years later, after the signs were removed, fishing from the balconies ceased.)

Dad told us at breakfast one day that he had been watching the seals from the balcony as they played in the surf. When we got back to the rooms, he pointed out the animals he had been watching. I saw that they were surfers in wet suits. Dad was sure that the surf was not high enough for surfing so they must be seals. The only other time he had seen surfing was in Hawaii, where the waves were five feet high.

Our realtor learned of a house that was not really on the market but the owners were considering selling. It was on the north side of Lake Madeline in Havre Lafitte. It had three bedrooms and a pool and was far better than anything we had seen, but still in our price range. It cost $75,000, and Dad thought it was too fancy for an assistant professor. He had built the house in Normal in 1947 for about $60,000 after fifteen years of practicing medicine and investing his income. Mom thought the house was just fine and helped us with the down payment.

When I started in Galveston, I was to be paid $45,000 per year. When I told Dad what I would be making, he was amazed. He told me that he was lucky to clear that much for a year of practice after he had been working for several years. He did not consider inflation or the level of my training. He had gone to work immediately after his internship during the Depression and later received six months of surgical residency.

We signed the papers on Thursday, but did not have a return flight until Sunday. Mom suggested that we go to San Antonio to visit Mrs. McGimpsey and Tanta (Aunt) Herta Koehler, Uncle Otto's niece. She made some phone calls, and we all headed for San Antonio in their car. We stayed at the historic St. Anthony's Hotel downtown. It had not been remodeled and came over as faded splendor.

Shortly after World War II, Brooks McGimpsey had a falling-out with Otto Koehler, the nephew. Brooks had been the financial genius behind the Pearl Brewery for years, but Otto was president of the brewery and wanted to run everything about the brewery so he fired Brooks and bought his interest in the brewery to get rid of him. Since then, the McGimpseys did not speak to the Koehlers and vice versa. Mom was on good terms with both, so we needed to see them each separately.

We met Mrs. McGimpsey and took her to lunch at a new restaurant she liked in an old colonial mansion in the north suburbs of San Antonio. We had a very nice lunch, and Dad and Mom had a wonderful time catching up with Mrs. McGimpsey. Mrs. Mac insisted that Scott try the mango ice cream that was one of the signature dishes of the restaurant. He took one bite and declared that he did not like it. The restaurant immediately substituted vanilla ice cream, which he loved.

After lunch, we took Mrs. Mac back to her house near Trinity College. We killed an hour driving around San Antonio before going to Tanta Herta's apartment. After chatting with Herta for several hours, she announced that she had made dinner reservations at a new restaurant in northern San Antonio—the same restaurant.

We took Scott aside to explain to him that Tanta Herta was not to know that we had been there with Mrs. McGimpsey so he should not mention that he had been to this restaurant before.

Fortunately, we were seated in a different part of the restaurant and had different wait staff. After dinner, Tanta Herta insisted that everyone have dessert and told Scott that he should try the mango ice cream. He told her that he did not like mango ice cream, but she was sure that he had never had it before. He told her that he had eaten mango ice cream and did not like it, but did not tell her where. Dad was impressed that a four-year-old boy did not blow it by revealing that we had eaten there for lunch with Mrs. McGimpsey.

My fellowship ended on June 30, 1973, but I delayed the start of my position in Galveston until September 1. I wanted to take some time in New England and have time to make an orderly move to Texas. I had to sell my sailboat, put the house in Marblehead on the market, and pack everything for the move to Galveston. It was going to cost more than the price of the sailboat to move it to Galveston so

I needed to sell it. I could not, in clear conscience, have the university pay for moving the sailboat.

My parents wanted to come to Marblehead and travel north through the Maritime provinces in Canada with us before we left New England. Right after they arrived in Marblehead, I took them out on my sailboat to watch the start of the Marblehead-to-Halifax sailboat race. We motored out to Tinker's Bell, the permanent buoy that was used for one end of the starting line. Motoring pleased Dad who was impatient with sailing. There were over a hundred boats milling around near the starting line, creating chaos. I decided to anchor near the start line and let them avoid me. As soon as we were anchored, the coast guard boat addressed the milling boats and ordered everyone to anchor. He used a megaphone to tell everyone to line up, side by side in a row, starting with my anchored sailboat. We had the perfect position to watch the start.

The racing sailboats ranged from thirty-five feet long to the large ocean racers of eighty to ninety feet. It was a downwind start. This created a danger of being pushed across the starting line before the starting gun, making them turn around and go back so they could cross the line again after the gun. If needed, this maneuver had to be done quickly so they did not want any extra sails to manage. Once the boats safely crossed the start line after the gun, they broke out the huge spinnaker sails for the downwind race. The boats were divided into classes by size. Each class started five minutes apart with the largest boats last. It was a glorious sight with almost one hundred boats flying colorful ballooning spinnakers.

They had two gray coast guard cutters to escort the fleet. Their job was to rescue boats in trouble and to chase off whales so they would not damage the sailboats. The fin keels, popular on the ocean racers, apparently excited the whales to rub against the boats, possibly damaging them. Dad wanted to get back home fast and Mom could not swim, so we motored back to the dock.

Several days later, we drove up through Maine to Bar Harbor and Cadillac Island. Mom got in an argument with the chef because he would not serve a lobster to Scott. The chef said he would not waste a lobster on a child because they would never eat it. Scott got his lobster and ate it. From there, we went to New Brunswick and on to Prince Edward Island for a few days. On the return, we went to Halifax and Peggy's Cove before taking the car ferry back to Maine.

When we arrived back in the United States, we had to go through customs. The customs inspector asked us if we had any firearms or firecrackers in the car. Scott was sitting in the backseat between Letha and his grandmother. He quickly volunteered that we had some crackers in the backseat, referring to the saltines they had been snacking on as the ferry unloaded.

At that point, we all had to get out of the car while they did a thorough inspection. Dad fussed and fumed the rest of the evening about Scott not being able to keep his mouth shut and the delay he had caused. Scott was about to have his fifth birthday and always wanted to be helpful. Dad had been in the army when Bruce and I were each four and five years old so he had not lived with a five-year-old and did not have much patience for Scott.

When Scott was four, Dad was left at home to babysit Scott and had to fix lunch for them. I was at work, and Letha and Mom had gone shopping. Dad put the milk carton on the table and got distracted with something. Scott attempted to pour the milk and managed to spill much of it on the table and the floor. Dad had to clean up the spilled milk from the table and kitchen floor. Scott's comment was that he was "just trying to help."

When we got back to Marblehead, Dad started having chest pain whenever he had to walk more than half a block. He had been riding in the car every day so it had not bothered him on the trip. I wanted him to get it checked in Boston, but he told me that he had an appointment with his doctor in Arkansas, as soon as he got home, and wanted to wait. They left a few days after the trip.

Marblehead was such a sailing town that I sold my Santana 21 sailboat in a few days. We packed up the house and loaded the moving van on August 16. Fortunately, UTMB was paying for our move to Texas so we did not have to discard very much.

Letha's aunt Mid came out from Pennsylvania to Marblehead to drive across country with us. We had two cars, so she entertained Scott while Letha drove in one car, I drove the other car. We all celebrated Scott's birthday, on August 18, with Letha's brother, Jim Foss, and his wife, Janice, in Columbus, Indiana, and again in Bull Shoals. We were racing the moving van to Galveston, so we had to be in Galveston by August twenty-first.

The van did not arrive until the twenty-sixth. When it did not arrive on the twenty-first as expected, we learned that the truck had lost its brakes on a hill in Connecticut. The driver rode out a long and fast ride downhill and managed to get the truck off the road and stopped on the uphill grade after reaching the bottom. He climbed out of the truck and hitchhiked into the next town. He called the company and told them to get another driver. He was not going to get into that truck again. It took several days for them to repair the truck and find another driver.

We moved in and unpacked in time for Tropical Storm Delia. The sustained winds officially hit seventy-four miles per hour so it was not an official hurricane with winds above seventy-five miles per hour. It came ashore just east of Galveston and dissipated. The weathermen lost track of the eye of the storm and assumed that it was over Louisiana.

The next day, the storm reformed over the gulf just southwest of Galveston and came through again. In the middle of the storm, the eye passed over our end of Galveston so we went out and stood in the sunshine by the overflowing swimming pool. The eye passed in about twenty minutes, and the wind and rain started again, as fierce as ever. We had plywood panels for hurricane shutters so we did not have any damage.

The day after the storm, Dad called to tell us that his doctor decided that he needed to have coronary bypass surgery. The doctor had recommended several places to go for the surgery. Two doctors on the list were Dr. Norman Shumway in San Francisco, where Bruce lived, and Dr. Denton Cooley in Houston, near where we lived. Since Bruce was a specialist in foreign trade and I was a doctor, Dad chose Houston so Mom could stay with us and he could recuperate in Galveston with my help. He asked me to call Dr. Cooley to make the arrangements.

Two weeks later, Mom and Dad drove from Bull Shoals to Galveston on Saturday. I took Dad down to show him my office on Sunday. The faculty saw our private patients in the private office building across the plaza from the hospital. The indigent clinic was in the hospital complex. Walking from the office building to the hospital, Dad had to stop twice to let his chest pain go away.

We took him to Methodist Hospital in Houston on Monday. Dr. Cooley explained that they would do a complete workup to decide if he was a good candidate for the surgery. Dad was seventy years old. Dr. Cooley had a general cutoff age, at that time, of sixty-five for *C*oronary *A*rtery *B*ypass *G*raft surgery (CABG). After the workup, Dr. Cooley said he would make an exception to his rule because Dad had been mowing the grass and chopping wood a few weeks before and was in great physical condition for a seventy-year-old.

After getting Dad to the hospital, I left immediately to attend the American Academy of Ophthalmology meeting in Dallas. I thought that they would not do surgery until Thursday or Friday or possibly the next week. On Tuesday, I was paged in the convention exhibit hall. The message at the paging desk was that Dad was scheduled for the first case on Wednesday morning. I should come to the hospital in Houston immediately. I checked out of the hotel, caught a plane back to Houston, and took a cab directly to the hospital Tuesday afternoon.

We had to be back at the hospital by 7:00 a.m. Wednesday if we wanted to see him before the surgery. We arranged for a neighbor to take care of Scott. Bruce and Judy had flown in from San Francisco and were staying at a hotel near the hospital. We all met at the hospital on Wednesday morning to go with Dad from his room as far as we could go to the operating room. Then we went to the waiting room. Dad was to be the first patient because he was the oldest patient that day. We sat in the waiting room all morning.

Dr. Cooley's nurse, dressed in scrubs, came out of the doors between the OR and the waiting room and talked with several families. She told them that the surgery was over and that they could see their loved one that evening during visiting hours. She did not talk with us. Mom was getting more and more upset with the wait.

Finally, a secretary came to the main doors of the waiting area and asked for the Barber family. We identified ourselves. She told us that Dr. Cooley wanted to speak with us in his office. Mom lost it. She was sure that Dr. Cooley wanted to personally tell us that Dad had died during surgery. She started crying and could hardly stand up. Bruce and I helped her up and walked her down the hall to the office.

After we were in the office area, Dr. Cooley came out of his inner office. He saw that my mother was crying and immediately assured her that everything had gone well. He explained that since my father was a doctor, he wanted to personally assure us that all was well and to invite the other doctors in the family, Letha and me, to come back that afternoon to watch bypass surgery from seats in the amphitheater. He told us that the doctors could come and go in the coronary ICU, but the rest of the family would have to wait until the evening visiting hours.

We took Mom to lunch before Letha and I went to the amphitheater to watch Dr. Cooley for a while and then visited Dad in the ICU. Mom stayed with Bruce and Judy. Dad was still out of it from the anesthesia, but resting well. We all stayed in Houston for evening visiting hours so Mom could see Dad.

Dad did very well for the first two days in the ICU. There were three ICUs with about twelve patients in each. The first ICU filled with Monday's patients, the second on Tuesday, and the third on Wednesday. The first ICU had to be emptied by Thursday morning for the next round of patients.

On the second day, Dad suffered a setback. The beds of the ICU were lined up on opposite walls with the feet of the beds facing each other. The patient across from Dad had a cardiac arrest, and the crash team did CPR. Dad, who was propped up in bed, watched the whole episode from his position across the room. The man did not recover and died as my father watched. Dad had lost patients in his practice and had seen people die, but watching someone die, who had just had the same operation that he had when he should have been getting better, was very depressing. Dad started having extra heartbeats, so they kept Dad in the ICU an extra day, until Saturday morning, before sending him to a monitored hospital floor.

Dad was amazed that they got him out of bed and had him walking around the halls of the monitored floor, leaning on his bed table as a walker, only two days after leaving the ICU. He did not have much pain after the first few days, but complained of feeling a crunch in his chest when he moved the wrong way. His sternum had been cut across to gain access to the heart. The bone was sewn back together with stainless steel wire sutures, but was loose enough that it shifted when he changed position.

He was sent home to our house about a week after surgery with instructions to walk around in the house several times a day for the next week. Then he was told to walk in the street (we did not have sidewalks) every day. At first, he would walk a block up the street and turn around and walk back. The block cross from us was three blocks long and one block wide with cul-de-sacs dividing the blocks, but not going all the way through the block. Every few days, he would add a block to his walk until he could walk the eight blocks around that section. Mom and Dad stayed with us until the weekend before Thanksgiving—more than two months.

Several weeks after returning to Arkansas, Dad started having a fever and chills. He was very worried that he had some kind of deep infection. I consulted Dr. Cooley and learned about "postpericardiotomy syndrome." People who have their chest and pericardium opened for heart surgery often develop fevers several months after surgery. Dr. Cooley had Dad take aspirin for a few days, and the fevers went away.

Chapter 30

Dad recovered from his bypass surgery and regained his usual activities in Bull Shoals. He mowed the grass, moved the boathouse, and fished with his buddies. He often talked about his fishing trips in Canada with Bruce and me. He decided that he wanted one more fishing trip to Lake of the Woods in Ontario. He called me to ask if we would go with him, saying that he thought he was too old to handle a boat by himself and carry outboard motors and other gear. We agreed to go with him. Mom decided to go on this trip, providing she did not have to fish. Letha and Scott, who was six, went with us, and they both wanted to fish.

Mom and Dad drove from Arkansas to International Falls and met us at the airport before crossing the border to Fort Francis, Ontario. We stayed at a different lodge than Bruce and Dad and I had stayed in when Dad took us to Sioux Narrows when I was in high school. Scott was only six and had not been fishing before so it was a great adventure for him. The first day, we took two boats with a guide for the four fishermen while Mom stayed at the lodge to read and take naps.

It was windy, making the water very rough the second day, so we decided to go up the river into another small lake to fish for bass and walleye. Since we would not be on a big lake, Mom decided to go with us and promised to pay for the mounting of any large fish that anyone caught. She was still mad at Dad for not bringing home and mounting the large northern pike I had caught on the Rainy Lake trip.

We did not have much success that day, so Mom and Dad went home early. Letha, Scott, and I were in a boat with Moses, our guide. Moses suggested that we fish for bass in the small river that connected two lakes. The bottom was gravel, and the water was so clear that the bottom was visible at a depth of about five feet.

We were using little red poppers with minnows for bait. Scott caught a bass that was about five inches long—too small to keep. As he reeled it in close to the boat, a muskie lunged for it at the surface. The muskie jumped out of the water and almost hit the side of the boat. Scott yanked the bass out of the water and was so proud of it. He wanted to keep it.

I told him to put it back in the water to see if the muskie would try to get it again. Scott hesitated but finally put the little bass into the water, and the muskie immediately went for it. This time, the muskie grabbed the fish and headed for the bottom. We could see the dark back of the fish hovering over the gravel bottom with the little red popper at one corner of its mouth. The tail of the bass was sticking out the other side.

I turned back the drag on Scott's reel while I told Scott to let the fish run with the bass until it stopped. I told Scott that once the fish stopped taking line, he should close the bail and yank the rod to set the hook.

The strategy worked as planned, and Scott had the muskie hooked. Moses immediately raised our anchor and tipped up the outboard motors so the fish could not get them tangled in the line. Scott fought the fish for about five minutes before he handed me his pole and insisted that I bring in the fish. He said it was too big for him.

Since we were not anchored, the boat drifted against the bank, and the raised motor snagged a small tree. Moses was afraid that being anchored to the bank would give the fish an advantage, so he pulled the tree out by its roots and threw it up on the bank. He pushed us off the bank and used a paddle to keep us away.

We fought the fish for about thirty minutes before we could get it alongside the boat. Moses netted it and threw it into the back corner of the boat where it flopped wildly for about thirty seconds. Boarding of the fish was accompanied by a round of applause and cheers. Our drama of fighting this big leaping fish had essentially closed the narrow river. Several boats heading in each direction had stopped to give us room and to watch us land the fish.

Moses threw a wet sack over the muskie to keep it quiet and wet and looked at his watch. It was almost five o'clock, and we had been talking about quitting and going home before we hooked the muskie. Moses said, "We quit! Go home! Fish dry out fast, lose weight."

Moses started the big motor, and we sped toward the lift-over dock. The Mando Paper Company was using the river to drift logs to the paper mill so there was a dam and sluice to lower them past a waterfall to the river below. The native Indians operated a lift-over service around the dam that consisted of a John Deere tractor and a wagon with a boat cradle.

There were several boats lined up at the dock, waiting for the lift-over. Moses stood up in the boat and waved to the tractor driver and pointed to a second dock. The driver went to the second dock to pick us up and lift us around the sluice, passing the other boats. I asked Moses how he managed to get us preference. He pointed to his chest and simply replied, "Me chief!"

As soon as we got to the dock, Moses grabbed the now-lifeless muskie and took it to the scale. It weighed twenty-three pounds and was forty-two inches long. The tip of the tail was touching the ground when it hung on the scale. Scott was so excited that he ran to tell his grandmother and grandfather. Dad was taking a nap, but Scott woke him up. Scott told him about the twenty-three-pound muskie, but Dad would not believe it. Scott dragged him out of bed and up to the scale to prove it. Dad was happy for Scott, but he kept muttering about fishing for muskie for years and never getting one in the boat, but this spoiled little kid had just caught a big one.

Mom said she would keep her promise to have it mounted although she thought it would have been a five-pound bass instead. We asked the staff at the lodge about taxidermists. They told us to take the muskie to the fish processing plant in the village so that they could flash freeze it overnight. We would have to take it about 160 miles to Winnipeg, Manitoba, to find a good taxidermist.

The fish processing plant had a blackboard where they posted large catches with the name of the fisherman. That night, we were in a gift shop looking around when someone asked Scott if he had been fishing. He shyly answered, "Yes."

They asked him if he caught anything and he answered, "Yes."

They asked him what he caught so he said, "I caught a big muskie."

They laughed. Then someone spoke up and said that the board at the fish house had posted a twenty-three-pound muskie caught by someone six years old.

The whole family took the next day off from fishing to take Scott's fish to Winnipeg. The people at the lodge gave us the name of a restaurant in Winnipeg where there were many mounted fish on the wall. These fish were all labeled by their taxidermist so we ate lunch there and studied the fish. We picked our favorite taxidermist from the examples there and were given directions to his shop. We carried the frozen fish into the shop where it was measured and put in the freezer.

We did not realize the complexity of mounting a fish. Scott had to decide whether he wanted it jumping up, fighting down, or straight, mouth open or closed. He first wanted it in the fighting down position with the open mouth and tail turned down, but when his grandmother asked him where he wanted to hang it, he told her that he wanted it over his bed. Dad asked him if he wanted to wake up looking at the big teeth in the open mouth of the muskie. Scott changed his mind to mouth open, fighting up.

Since this big fish had been caught on a little red popper, we had them put the popper in the corner of the fish's mouth as it had been when we caught it. When he caught the fish, there was no leader attached to the lure; the popper was tied to the six-pound test nylon line. It was a miracle that the big teeth on the muskie had not cut the line.

The taxidermist had a backlog of fish and several big rattlesnakes to mount so it would be several months until they shipped the muskie to us in Texas.

We had several more days of fishing for walleye, so Dad had a relaxed time fishing without having to run the motors or carry the gear. He had time to show Scott how he could tie knots and handle instruments without his left thumb, just as he had shown Bruce and me years before. We caught enough fish so Dad was able to ship fish home and they could have a fish fry for their friends back home in Arkansas.

In early October, Letha received a call from the bus station in Galveston to pick up a crate from Winnipeg. After she picked up Scott from school, they went to the bus station, paid for the shipment, and loaded a large wooden box into the backseat of the car.

On the way home, Scott asked his mother not to be upset, but he was sure that they had sent the wrong fish. The fish was still in the box so she knew that he could not see it. She asked him why he thought they had sent the wrong fish. He replied that they had sent a codfish instead of the muskie. Scott knew about codfish from living in New England. Letha asked him why he thought it was a codfish. He told her that it was written on the box and pointed to where it said C.O.D. on the box. When we pried open the box at home, it had the big muskie inside.

The fishing trip was such a success that Mom soon proposed another trip. Dad was a big fan of the *Huntley-Brinkley Report*. Chet Huntley would occasionally talk about his "Big Sky Ranch" in Montana. They had built a hotel on the ranch and turned it into a dude ranch. Dad wanted to see the ranch, but did not want to do all the driving to get there, especially in the mountains. We agreed to fly to meet them at Rapid City, South Dakota, to take over the driving from there.

We visited Mount Rushmore and the Crazy Horse monument near Rapid City. Dad got to talk with Korczak Ziolkowski, the man who was blasting the mountain to reveal the statue of Crazy Horse. Ziolkowski explained the work ahead to blast away most of a mountain to create a huge statue of an Indian on horseback.

We drove on to spend a few days in the Tetons before moving on to Yellowstone. This was the first time Scott had seen the Rocky Mountains, bison, or elk. Dad was in his element explaining all this to Scott.

From Yellowstone, it was on to the highlight of the trip, Huntley's Big Sky Ranch. Dad said he was too old to ride a horse and told us again that he had ridden a horse to school many times when he was growing up. Letha, Scott, and I went for a trail ride while Mom and Dad relaxed at the ranch.

Letha had jeans, a western-cut shirt, cowboy boots, and a Stetson hat to wear riding. When the wrangler saw her, he asked if she could ride. We had ridden horses at dude ranches so she said yes. The wrangler commented that Mrs. Huntley's horse had not been ridden for several days so it would be good for Letha to ride her horse. It happened that Mrs. Huntley's horse was a very spirited horse that wanted to jump all the little streams and gallop in the open. Letha was not ready for that type of horse, so eventually the wrangler had to walk beside her to lead her horse by the bridle to keep the horse from throwing Letha.

From Big Sky we crossed Southwest Montana into Idaho. It snowed in the mountains that morning on the Fourth of July, while we followed the Salmon River along the Sawtooth Mountains to reach Salmon, Idaho. Dad said that he had never been snowed upon on the Fourth of July, even when he was in Greenland.

Going on south in Idaho, we saw the Twin Falls of the Snake River and dropped down to Jackpot, Nevada. Scott saw his first casino there because we had to walk through it to get to the hotel dining room for lunch. Dad told Scott what he had told me many times: "If you want to double your money, simply fold it over and put it back in your pocket." Dad did not believe in gambling for anything more than pennies. He said that he had worked too hard for his money to risk it gambling.

The next major stop was Vail, Colorado. Letha and I had taken Scott there to ski in the winter, but Mom and Dad had never seen Vail. Dad had not skied since he twisted his knee in Greenland, but it was summer so Vail was full of hikers, mountain climbers, and tennis players. We stayed at the Vail Lodge, which Dad thought was pretty ritzy.

    Mom and Dad put us on a plane in Denver for the flight to Texas and then drove back to Arkansas. Letha, Scott, and I had such a great time that we did a similar trip the next summer with Letha's family and returned the following year by ourselves.

Chapter 31

After fourteen years in Arkansas, Mom and Dad had a circle of friends including fourteen couples who socialized and explored Arkansas together. The men picked berries, hunted, and fished together. The wives played cards and helped each other cope with the difficult living in northern Arkansas. Couples would get together for a day trip to see an old ferry or a mining ghost town. The group had parties about once a month.

Suddenly, within one year, one member of each couple died, except my parents. The surviving spouse of each couple soon moved back to the area where they had lived before moving to Arkansas. This was to be near family or for better medical care. The new people who were moving into the area were about ten to fifteen years younger than my parents and were new to the area so they wanted to do things that were old experiences to my parents.

Life in Arkansas was difficult. They had to go to the post office for mail. The nearest full grocery store and other shopping were fifteen miles away in Mountain Home. The boathouse had to be moved every time the level of the lake changed, which was often, because the lake was used for power generation. They decided to try out Arizona for retirement living, so they sold the house in Arkansas and headed for the Phoenix area.

After one winter of renting an apartment at a motel in Mesa, Arizona, they decided to locate in Mesa. They found a two-bedroom apartment with a south-facing patio that overlooked a nine-hole executive golf course. When the irrigation sprays came on in the evening, Mom would say that the fountains were playing for the cocktail hour. The backdrop of the view from the patio was San Tan Mountain, about fifteen miles away.

There was a shortage of rental apartments for the winter demand so all apartments were rented for the entire year or not at all. When Scott did several summers at Arizona State University in Tempe, we would stay in the apartment for a few days when we took him to the program and picked him up. He was in the gifted and talented program for eighth-grade students at Arizona State University. After qualifying on the SAT exam in seventh grade, they could take various college courses and study high school mathematics during the summer.

After my parents moved to Phoenix, my father continued to have medical problems. He continued to have prostate symptoms, causing him to undergo a TUR (transurethral resection) about every three or four years. While we lived in Galveston, I hooked him up with Dr. Michael Warren who was chief of Urology at UTMB. Mike did an uneventful TUR and sent my father on his way a few days later. I ran into Mike in the doctor's lounge in the operating room about a week later. He told me that the tissue removed from my father was found to have cancer in it. He said I should tell my father.

I asked Mike to call my father to tell him so that he could answer my father's questions since I did not know much about the current treatment of prostate cancer. He told me that there was not much to be done and that my father would die of something else before the prostate cancer got him. I told Mike that he was my father's doctor so he should tell him about his cancer. I managed to shame him into calling my father because this conversation was held in front of several other doctors in the lounge.

Dad contacted a urologist in Phoenix who put him on hormone suppression therapy. He did well for a while, but would eventually develop obstructive symptoms and still had to have repeat TURs every three years.

After the move to Phoenix, they found that it was too hot in the summer, so they would spend the summer months in Illinois. They bought a small house in the north end of Normal. Dad would grow tomatoes and red raspberries in the backyard. They had way too many tomatoes so he tried to give them away.

All their neighbors also grew tomatoes, so every morning, he would run into several of the neighbors who would be out walking the neighborhood with buckets of tomatoes trying to give them away. He was the only one in the neighborhood who grew raspberries so he did not have difficulty giving them away.

One night, I received a frantic call from my mother who was in Illinois. She was in Brokaw Hospital and was very upset. Dr. Stutsman had found a lump in her breast, and Dr. Hoopes had done a biopsy the day before. She had developed a hematoma at the biopsy site that was very painful. She told me that the doctors wanted to reoperate to remove the hematoma. Mom was raised a Christian Scientist and had been healthy to this point except for migraine headaches and bouts of depression. She thought the surgeon had made an error and caused the hematoma, so she was reluctant to let him try again.

Dr. Hoopes had been a close friend and fellow surgeon of Dad's for many years, and Dad had the utmost confidence in him. My mother thought that friendship was behind my father's support of Dr. Hoopes so she would not agree to the intervention.

I talked with her for about an hour, explaining that it was a recognized complication and that it was best treated by surgical drainage rather than waiting for weeks for it to absorb. She was not convinced, so I flew to Bloomington and went to the hospital to talk with her. Meanwhile, the biopsy report had come back as a nonmalignant fibroma. After about half an hour of explanations, she agreed to have the hematoma drained. It was done the next day, and the pain was relieved. It went on to heal without recurrence of the hematoma.

August in Illinois was usually very hot—too hot for my mother. They started renting an apartment for that month in the highlands of Colorado near Gunnison. Mom could sit on the balcony and read while Dad fished the lesser streams that emptied into the Gunnison River before the Black Canyon. He talked with the local people for advice and went to ranches to ask permission. He had "never met a stranger" so he usually got permission. Having grown up on the farm, he always closed gates and was careful where he drove. When he fished these streams, he would always catch and release the trout he caught. He did not have his smoker, and Mom did not want to cook them. He often found other fishermen to go with him because some of the streams were fast enough to be dangerous.

After he retired, his illnesses did not slow him down. He and Mom continued to live an active life and travel the world. They went to Australia and New Zealand and spent several days in the mountains of New Zealand fishing for trout. They told me that their guide was the guide who took the Queen of England fishing when she visited New Zealand. The fishing was excellent, but the guide insisted that they stop every afternoon to brew "Billy Tea."

They took several trips to Europe, made an extensive trip to China, and toured the South Pacific where my father purchased a

Fiji Island coconut shredder, which he enjoyed using until he died. About 1980, Dad decided that he had seen the world and that there was no place like "the Good Old USA" so he gave up traveling. Air travel had gotten to be too much of a hassle for him.

With the move to Phoenix, Dad had to find new hobbies to replace the hunting and fishing of the Ozarks. The community they lived in was designed for retired people. The community center had a metal shop, a wood shop, and a lapidary shop for the men. For the women, there were rooms for sewing, crafts, and playing cards. Outside, there were bocce courts, tennis courts, and an eighteen-hole golf course.

Dad decided to take up lapidary work. He could go in the morning and put fifty cents in the maintenance fund box to allow him to use any of the saws and grinders. There were several men who were experienced who served as proctors and instructors. He started with cutting and polishing stones for jewelry. At first, he did mostly agate and local rocks, but he soon moved on to tiger eye, malachite, and jade.

He had a canvas carry-on bag that he kept his work in so he could grab his bag at about nine o'clock in the morning and head for the rock shop and his lapidary buddies. He would be home at noon for lunch. In the afternoon, he often played bocce with some of his friends and went to the community pool to swim and relax in the sun.

He started with small stones that he made into pendants and the clasps for bolo ties. In Arizona, everyone wore bolo ties. Usually he would cut the stones and hone them into various shapes before polishing them to a fine finish. He would present them to his friends, but he would never sell them. He always said that his work was so good "it was priceless." After about one hundred pendants and bolo ties, he started doing stone spheres and bookends. He would cut and shape the stones and polish the dress faces. He would sign and date his works on the back or bottom with a black felt pen.

When he had all the bookends he could use or give away, he started making clocks from slabs of agate or other stones. He used a special drill bit to cut round holes in the middle of the slab to fit it with a battery-powered clock mechanism. These stones would be finished to a smooth dull finish. If water was sprayed on the rock, the colors became vivid and the surface was shiny smooth. As soon as the water dried, the surface became dull and the colors faded. To keep the shine and colors, he would coat the rock with polyurethane. This took skill to keep from having bubbles or brush strokes in the polyurethane. Once the coating was dry, he would apply numbers or markers to make the clock face and install the mechanism and hands. He gave clocks to friends and family and had several scattered around the house. He donated several of these clocks to the Brokaw Hospital gift shop to sell to raise money for the hospital auxiliary.

I now have several clocks, six pairs of bookends, about twenty bolo ties, and two perfect agate spheres. Judy and my daughter-in-law, Sheena, have many of the pendants and earrings including green and black jade, gold and blue tiger eye, malachite, lapis, and fossils. When he was particularly proud of a jewelry stone, he would take it to a friend at Apache Junction who would band it with gold or sterling silver.

Dad loved the desert and soon learned the names of most of the cacti and dessert flowers. He and Mom would go for walks and look for desert quail and cactus wrens. The area was too densely populated for there to be many poisonous snakes. In their neighborhood, there was a hundred-foot-wide swath of undeveloped desert under some power lines. There was a well-traveled path that made for easy walking.

The Phoenix area was full of rock hounds, so there were frequent rock shows and rock sales. Pickup trucks with rock exhibits on the tailgates would line the old abandoned runways at Luke Air Force Base at least once each year.

One time, Dad took us to Bee Creek, north of Phoenix, to visit the man who was the source of lizard stone, a green rock with white lizard-shaped patterns throughout the stone. That man also had a gold sluice in his backyard that he used to recover gold from stone and gravel that he brought from his claim. He told us that he always went by a different route to mine his claim in the mountains to prevent claim jumpers from learning its location. He showed us some large nuggets he had found there.

Dad and Mom would go for long rides on roads through the desert. They could name all the local mountain peaks. Dad always liked to explore new places and tell other people about them. I must have inherited my love of exploring from Dad.

Chapter 32

About seven years after his bypass surgery, Dad ran across an article in a medical journal that was a report of survival rates after coronary artery bypass graft surgery in Veterans Administration hospitals. The results showed that the mean survival after CABG (pronounced cabbage) surgery was five years. He called me to tell me that he was living on borrowed time since it had been more than five years since his surgery.

I asked one of the thoracic surgeons in Galveston what he thought was the mean survival after CABG surgery. He said upward of ten years. I went to the library to research survival rates and found several reports of mean survival that ranged from greater than five years to near ten years with many people surviving longer.

I told Dad about these other reports and explained that the VA system usually had the poorest results of anyone, but he had a copy of the VA article with the data and would not believe me. When I visited at Christmas, he gave me several of the medical books he had saved, saying that I should take them because he would die soon. He also gave me one of his old stethoscopes and some of the surgical instruments he had saved from his practice to use for tying flies for fishing and working with his stone jewelry. He lived for six years after reading that report and died from complications of his prostate cancer, proving Dr. Warren wrong.

In about 1980, Mom had some abnormal bleeding and stopped in Galveston on the way back to Normal in the spring. Dr. William McGanity, the chairman of the ob-gyn department, did a biopsy that showed endometrial cancer. Mom and Dad stayed in one of our rental condos for two months while she had a hysterectomy and recovered sufficiently for radiation therapy. Node dissection did not detect any metastases, but Dr. McGanity recommended "a light dusting" of radiation in case they had missed a positive lymph node.

When Dad visited her in the hospital in the evenings, he would stay until the end of visiting hours. Mom would call home to tell us when he left with instructions to go look for him if he did not arrive home in fifteen minutes. Dad never got lost. Mom told us that we should not tell Dad that she worried about him.

When she was discharged from the hospital, Dad was promoted to nurse. He looked after Mom as she recovered from the surgery and got back on her feet. For the first week or so, he was very attentive and took very good care of her. As she became ambulatory, he let her do more and more until he became bored.

Dad was always restless when he was away from home and did not have his usual ways to fill his time. He became a nuisance around the house and always wanted something to do. He could not find a rock hound club in Galveston, but I knew that Truman Blocker, the retired president of UTMB, had a garage full of rocks that he had collected from around the world. I managed to introduce Dad to Dr. Blocker. They had both been army surgeons in World War II and had many stories to swap. Dr. Blocker took Dad to rock shows in Houston and introduced him to several other rock hounds in the Galveston area.

Dr. Blocker had bad knees so he walked with a cane. Because of the cane, Dad referred to him as "the Old Doctor" although I was sure that Dr. Blocker was several years younger than Dad.

Truman Blocker was a plastic surgeon who was Dan Blocker's older bigger brother. (Dan Blocker played Hoss Cartwright in *Bonanza* on TV until he died after gallbladder surgery in a Los Angeles hospital.) Dr. Blocker wore size 9 (extra large) gloves when he operated, but did very delicate plastic surgery specializing in burn repairs.

Truman was a very gregarious person and had been a good fundraiser for the university. There were many stories about him. Once, when the University of Texas sent a private plane to Galveston to bring him to a meeting at the main campus in Austin, he asked for some bourbon when he boarded. The attendant told him that the bar could not open until they reached ten thousand feet. As soon as they took off, Dr. Blocker slid down low in his seat and looked out the window. He told the attendant that he could not see the ground so they must be over ten thousand feet. He got his bourbon.

He gained fame for his management of the medical team during the Texas City disaster in 1947 when a ship loaded with ammonium nitrate fertilizer blew up during repairs at the dock. Parts of the ship were found almost two miles from the scene of the explosion. Dr. Blocker activated his army hospital team, most of whom had come home to the medical branch in Galveston. They triaged the injured survivors and managed to save many lives.)

Mom was waiting for sufficient postsurgical healing so that she could start radiation. She was ready to start radiation when she developed an unusual hernia that had to be surgically repaired. This postponed the radiation therapy another six weeks until the new surgery had healed. They were tired of living in my condo in

Galveston and a hot summer was coming, so they decided to go back to Illinois for the radiation.

Dad took Mom to see Dr. Stutsman again. Dr. Stutzman sent my mother to Peoria, fifty miles away, for the radiation. Although Dr. McGanity in Galveston had recommended "a dusting of radiation" in case there was a positive lymph node from the cancer, the oncologist in Peoria gave her maximum radiation including a radium implant and multiple X-ray treatments. She was sick the whole summer from radiation sickness and did not feel better until several months after they had returned to Phoenix for the winter.

Letha, Scott, and I went to Normal during the time when Mom was getting her radiation. She was very ill from radiation sickness that had caused chronic diarrhea. Dad was trying to get ready to close and sell the house in Normal. He said that Bruce had shown very little interest in his collection of Eskimo artifacts and wanted to know if I was interested. Scott had always liked the polar bear rug, so Dad wanted to give it to him. Scott was glad to have it.

I had read most of Dad's Arctic books and always admired the kayaks and dolls in the collection. I told him I wanted the collection when he no longer had use for it. He packed it up and sent everything to me. The collection was in beautiful condition. We were adding a second floor to our house in Galveston, so when our architect learned of the collection, she designed a three-panel display case at the top of the stairs to show the collection.

When we took Scott to New England to look at colleges, I took photographs of the collection and made a visit to the Robert Perry Museum at Bowdoin College in Brunswick, Maine. I made an appointment to show them to the curator to see if they were interested in donations. When we arrived for the appointment, the assistant curator met me instead. She showed no interest in the items, saying, condescendingly, they had better and did not need more. I went through the museum and did not see anything of the quality and preservation of Dad's collection.

Dad's collection consisted of an assortment of items. There were two eiderdown baby blankets, one plain and one embroidered with the colorful green, black, and white head feathers of the eider duck. The eiderdown is so soft that it is difficult to tell exactly when you touch it. There were several pairs of sealskin mukluks varying from daily-wear fur slippers to fancy leather wedding boots. There are two kayaks made from bones and seal skin with miniature wood and ivory spears, harpoons, and paddles. The kayaks are about fifteen inches long, and both have carved and costumed Eskimo figures in them. There are several ivory forks and knives and carved walrus ivory Eskimo figures. There are two dolls that are clothed in furs. One is holding a skin drum; the other is a woman with a papoose holding a baby doll on her back. They are ten and fourteen inches tall respectively.

There is an ivory dogsled with dogs in harness and several small animal carvings. The Eskimo women wove beaded doilies with multicolored beads, and they adorned their clothes with these beads and dyed leather. Dad was given three of these doilies and a belt decorated with colored leather and beads.

One of his prize gifts was a carved Eskimo head, about six inches tall that was carved from driftwood. Driftwood is very scarce in Greenland. Since there are no native trees, it is considered very valuable.

Many of the books that Mom collected in Boston shortly after World War II are now out of print. The collection is now on display in the living room of our home and will probably go to the Carnegie Museum of Pittsburgh if Scott does not want it.

On the way back to Phoenix in the fall, a year later, Mom stopped in Galveston to see Dr. McGanity for follow up on her uterine cancer. He did routine lab work and did not expect to find anything. To save his patients money, Dr. McGanity sent his entire laboratory testing out of town. My parents left for Phoenix two days after her appointment. Dr. McGanity called me several days later to tell me that the lab tests had shown a very high white blood cell count, probably meaning that she had developed leukemia.

Knowing that radiation has long been linked to cancer, I often wonder if her leukemia was related to her massive radiation for her endometrial cancer. Most of the doctors I have asked about this think that the time interval between the radiation and the onset of leukemia was too short.

I talked to the top leukemia expert in Galveston to see what should be done. He said she needed a workup to confirm the diagnosis and to learn more about the type of leukemia that she had to be able to determine the type of therapy she needed. The leukemia expert in Galveston had trained a hematology oncologist several years before who was now practicing in Phoenix. He called the Phoenix doctor and made the referral.

I called Dad and gave him the name of the doctor so he could set up an appointment. They went to see the doctor. Dad took an immediate dislike to the doctor because he wore a full beard, was brusque, and was Jewish. My father thought that any doctor who did surgery or worked with immune-compromised patients should not have facial hair because of an increased risk of infection. He later referred to the doctor as "that fuzzy-faced Jew."

The doctor drew blood and did a bone marrow aspiration from the rim of Mom's pelvic bone. My mother claimed that he did not use anesthetic, or at least it did not work, so she had a great deal of pain that was made worse by the doctor's rough manner. After they left the doctor's office, she told Dad that she would never go back to that doctor. Dad was not impressed with the doctor and did not argue with her.

They managed to find another hematologic oncologist through their general doctor. He started her on chemotherapy, which she tolerated better than the massive radiation that she had received in Illinois. Her white blood cell count dropped but still had leukemic cells, which meant that she was suppressed, but not in remission.

When it was time to go to Illinois in the spring, she was still on therapeutic doses of chemotherapy, but her white count was down. The doctor in Phoenix transferred her care to Dr. Stutzman in Normal with instructions concerning the change from therapeutic to maintenance therapy if she went into remission.

Dr. Stutzman decided that her low white count meant that she was in remission and switched her to maintenance therapy. By the end of the summer, she was having severe pains in her legs and arms and her white blood count was sky-high. She was developing a "packed marrow syndrome." She had so many leukemia cells that her bone marrow was stuffed with white cells, making her bones ache. Mom and Dad sold the house in Normal, and Dad got her back out to Phoenix by car. The doctor in Phoenix put her back on therapeutic doses, and she responded some.

Chapter 33

My parents had been renting for several years in Mesa and had decided to buy a house there. We had taken Scott to the ASU program again that summer and spent a week in Phoenix. Mom had asked us to contact a realtor and have her watch for a house on a golf course with a south-facing patio for the winter sun. Mesa is so flat that the mountains disappear behind the house across the street unless there is an open view across something like a golf course.

When they arrived, they contacted the realtor and spent several days with her looking at houses. They found one on a golf course with an east-facing patio and bought it. It was a two-bedroom house with a double garage and a nice kitchen. It was not furnished so they would have to furnish it before they could move in.

From the patio, they could see Red Mountain to the north, San Tan Mountain to the south, and Superstition Mountain to the east. They could sit on their patio to watch the golfers play past. The windows were screened to protect them from stray golf balls. Dad would pick up several golf balls in their backyard every evening.

By the time they had bought the house, Mom was worn out and took to her bed back at the apartment. She told me she did not have the energy to furnish the house so they could move into it. She thought she was going to die before they could move in.

I called Bruce and apprised him of the situation. Bruce and Judy and Letha, Scott, and I all met at the apartment in the Mesa suburb of Phoenix on the first weekend in November. Mom was convinced that she might die in the next few days, but she wanted to move into the house before she did. She was worried that Dad would not move into the house after she died, but she wanted him to live there. We made arrangements to return the next week to furnish the house so they could move in.

Armed with Mom's credit cards, we charged the department stores. We outfitted the kitchen from towels to stainless dinnerware, pots and pans, and basic foods. We went to two rental furniture stores to rent beds, sofas, recliners, TV, etc., to fill the house. We convinced the stores to deliver the furniture immediately because of Mom's condition. We spent a day in the house making the beds, setting up the kitchen, and trying to make it look homey. Dad was staying at the apartment with Mom while we did this.

When all was ready, we went to the apartment to get Mom. She was up and in a wheelchair but refused to go to the house. She said she was sure that she was going to die that day and did not want to die on the way to the house. Dad, Bruce, and I all tried to convince her that she was not going to die right away and that the house was ready. She held out until after it was dark and then agreed to go to the house. We learned later that she did not want to be seen by the neighbors as she left and have to "say goodbye" to them.

We managed to get her from her wheelchair in to the car while it was in the carport. We drove into the garage at the house and got her back into her wheelchair. Dad wheeled her through the house to show her how it was furnished and decorated and then put her to bed in the front bedroom.

Letha had come back to Mesa prepared to care for her until she died. Letha slept in the other twin bed in Mom's room. Dad was in the king-sized bed in the master bedroom. Bruce stayed and slept on the sleeper couch in the family room. Judy went back to San Francisco, and Scott and I went back to Galveston the next day.

Scott went back to school, and I had my usual routine at work. Scott and I would fly to Phoenix every weekend. Since I was chairman of the department, I did not take night or weekend call so it was easy for me to get away.

We got to know the stewardesses on Republic Air. They would tell us what was for dinner when we boarded the plane. Letha would come to the airport to pick us up and we would go to Scottsdale for lunch before going to the house. This was Letha's only time-out of the house each week. Letha stayed with Mom while Dad did the grocery shopping, and Dad looked after Mom while Letha was gone to the airport.

Bruce had learned that my grandfather's trust would expire on January 1 and the principal would be owned directly by my mother if she was still alive. The corpus of the trust would then go to my father when she died and be depleted by inheritance tax. If he did not spend it, Bruce and I would inherit it when he died, but have to pay inheritance taxes again. It would be taxed twice. If Mom died before January 1, the corpus was to be divided between Bruce and me and would not be taxed again after my grandfather's inheritance tax paid twenty-five years before.

Mom was telling Bruce that she was in pain and wanted to die. Dad, Letha, and I, being doctors, were against assisted death and would allow whatever happened to the inheritance to occur. Dad was worried that Bruce might assist Mom in her death. Dad had told Letha not to leave Mom at home alone with Bruce. Letha would stay in the house whenever Dad went out.

We had Thanksgiving in the house with the whole family there. We brought Mom to the table, but she only ate a few bites and wanted to go back to bed.

Scott and I continued to fly to Phoenix every weekend. Economy seats were $199; first-class seats were $299. Last-minute seats on economy were $299, and first-class tickets were $300. Because of the stress we were under and the day-to-day expectations preventing us from long-term planning, we usually flew first-class—out Friday night or Saturday morning, back Sunday night.

Mom was asking for pain medicine every few hours. I asked her doctor to prescribe longer-acting Dilaudid for her. He told me that none of the pharmacies would stock Dilaudid and that the hospital would not dispense it for outpatient use. He finally found a pharmacy that would dispense it on prescription, but the pharmacy was twenty miles away, in Tempe.

I took the prescription to the pharmacy. The outside windows were covered with woven-steel barriers. The pharmacy counter was walled off with thick bulletproof glass. There was a bank-teller-type drawer for transactions. They filled the prescription in less than five minutes, and it only cost about eight dollars for twenty pills. I commented to the pharmacist that I thought it was very inexpensive. He responded that legal heroin was cheap, but I could probably pay off the mortgage with what might be left over by selling it on the street.

Mom refused the Dilaudid, saying that she thought it would be too strong and she did not want to be drugged. I think her upbringing as a Christian Scientist had a lot to do with her decision. At the end, she did complain of severe pain, so she finally took a few of the Dilaudid when Letha offered it to her the day before she died. I think that I had let it slip that Dilaudid was actually heroin, which might have influenced her avoidance.

On my last visit with Mom, she told me that I should look after Dad. She thought he would have difficulty living alone and might have to move in with Letha and me. She knew that Dad would never live with Bruce and Judy. She said that he would be hard to live with because he was so stubborn and opinionated.

She also told me that she had always blamed Dad for Bruce's illnesses. She thought that Dad's pressure on Bruce had caused his ulcerative colitis although Dad would never accept the common theory that his ulcerative colitis was caused by stress. She also blamed Dad's arthritis genes for Bruce's other diseases.

Mom told me that she and Dad were proud of the way Bruce and I had made successful lives. She knew that Dad had told Bruce many times that he needed a master's degree in business (an MBA) if he wanted to rise to the top of his field, but that Bruce had always refused more schooling. He thought his certificate from Thunderbird in Phoenix was the equivalent of an MBA, but learned that his bosses did not give it that much weight.

Letha called me in the morning, on December 21, to tell me that Mom had died during the night. Dad's medical experience told him that she was dying, so he said goodbye to her at about midnight. Letha had been up with her all night trying to soothe her so Dad did not have to see her die. Scott was to be out of school for the Christmas break, so we flew to Phoenix immediately.

Mom and Dad attended a Presbyterian Church in Mesa. Dad arranged a memorial service with the minister there after Christmas. They had several friends from Normal who wintered in the Phoenix area, and there were several local friends in attendance. Mom's wish was to be cremated and have her ashes scattered on Red Mountain.

It was her favorite rock formation, and she could see it from the patio of their new house.

Bruce found a pilot at the Mesa Airport who made gas money for his plane by dropping cremated remains at selected spots. We learned that there were no restrictions about scattering ashes in Arizona, so we hired him to drop Mom's ashes in the notch of Red Mountain.

The day after the memorial service, Lee Long led a short sunrise memorial service, with scripture and prayer, for a group of us who gathered in a park on the banks of the Verde River. The Longs, Oars, and Kuchans, longtime friends from Normal, were there with some of her Mesa friends. As we watched, a lone plane flew out of the west and circled Red Mountain once before flying directly over the mountain. There was a cloud of dust from the tail of the plane that dissipated before landing on the mountain, but we were all sure that it settled in the notch, where she wanted. She had picked a giant and very permanent grave marker.

Dad settled in at the new house. They had been there a little more than one month, but he felt at home. He went back to his lapidary work and kept in touch with his local friends. Mom and Dad had been married only two months less than fifty years, but Dad said he had no desire to marry again.

He would invite various friends in for breakfast on Sunday mornings. He loved buckwheat pancakes and they were easy to fix. After several months, some of his friends called me to ask if I could intervene and get him to fix something else for breakfast.

They loved to go to his house on Sunday mornings. He was always entertaining with his many stories and jokes and they liked to be with him, but the buckwheat pancakes felt like lead in their stomachs and made them feel bad all day. He would not give up the buckwheat pancakes, but I convinced him to combine the batter half and half with light pancake mix. Everyone agreed it was much better.

Because Mom died before January 1, 1984, the trust did pass to Bruce and to me. Dad was upset about this. He had worked hard as a doctor and saved some money and made good investments. Mom had inherited her money. Before her inheritance, Dad's accountant had convinced him to divide his money and put half of it in Mom's name. This was in case he was sued for malpractice and was cleaned out by the lawsuit. When Mom inherited her money, she could not give any of it to Dad because most of it was in trust, but she used some of it to set up the trusts for Bruce and me. Dad always felt slighted by this.

They had a joint trust fund from Dad's money that paid them enough to live comfortably. Mom usually paid for their extensive travel from her trust. They lived in nice houses, drove the cars they wanted, and did not deny themselves anything they really wanted. Dad still had the joint trust fund that had over two hundred and fifty thousand dollars in investments from which he received a monthly payment from the income. When I visited him, he always complained that he did not have the money he should have. I tried to take him shopping for clothes, but he said he did not need any more clothes. He did not want to travel abroad and had money to fly anywhere he wanted in the United States. He was not spending everything he got from the trust, so every time we talked about this, his bank account had more money than the time before.

Several months after Mom died, he went to San Francisco to visit Bruce and Judy. He stayed for about two weeks. He told me that Judy started ignoring him and he began to feel that he was in the way, so he came back to Mesa to be among his friends. He started walking a mile a day for exercise. Mesa was flat as a floor, and he felt it made his knees feel better. He could cook well enough to take care of himself and occasionally ate out. He liked Marie Calendar's cafeteria, especially the pies.

When I went out to Mesa that spring to help him with his income taxes, he expressed a worry that since he lived alone, he might have a heart attack and not be able to summon help or he might die and not be found for several days. He said the neighbors across the street were willing to check on him, but he did not know them very well and did not want to impose on them.

St. Mary's Hospital in Galveston had just started a daily check-in program for people living alone. I called the local hospitals in Mesa, but they did not have a program like that. I called several local alarm companies in Mesa, but they were not interested until I found an owner who had just returned from an alarm convention where these systems were discussed. I convinced him to make my father his first customer. Within a year, people monitoring had become a major part of his business.

The alarm company installed a button in Dad's bathroom that he was to push at least once in twenty-four hours to keep them from sending the EMS people. He also had a panic button on a lanyard that he was to wear around his neck, but he seldom wore it. Dad decided to push the bathroom button when he got ready for bed at night. Since Dad went to bed at different times, he had several home emergency calls when he stayed up late. A couple of times, he forgot to push the button and was awakened by the EMS people.

The people across the street had the key to his front door and would let the EMS people in. Dad wore hearing aids that he took out at night and could not hear the phone or the EMS people pounding on the door once he went to bed. We convinced him to push the button morning and night, and that ended the emergency calls.

As far as I know, he never developed a close friendship with any women after Mom died. The Longs and the Kuchans had moved to Mesa and looked after him, included him in their parties, and took him to lunch occasionally. He had men friends that he walked with when he did his mile walk or worked with him in the lapidary shop.

Chapter 34

In October 1986, when Bruce was forty-nine years old, he began feeling weak and became slightly jaundiced. He was having fever and chills and periods of overwhelming weakness and jaundice. This time, his doctors did a liver biopsy and diagnosed cholangiocarcinoma of the liver (cancer of the bile ducts in the liver). Abscesses that developed behind the cancer-blocked bile ducts were giving him sepsis with fever. He told Dad, so Dad called me to find out what I knew about this rare cancer. I had to look it up and could not learn much about it except the definition.

I consulted some of my surgical and oncology friends in Galveston who told me that it was a bad actor. There was no known successful treatment. Radiation was ineffective. Chemotherapy was hit or miss. The usual time from diagnosis to death was about three months, regardless of treatment.

One of the oncologists at Stanford was using chemotherapy agents labeled with antibodies to the tumor to attract the chemotherapy agents to the tumors, but they declined to try it on Bruce because of his prior pulmonary disease, which appeared to be caused by his immune system.

Bruce was referred to a radiation oncologist who told him that he had a new protocol that would give him up to a year of "quality time." He convinced Bruce to donate $10,000 to his research as part of his therapy. Bruce started the radiation, but continued to have bouts of sepsis and abdominal pain. His doctor, who had been his allergist, now proclaimed himself an oncologist who could manage this illness.

Bruce told me his real doctor "hero" was the intervention radiologist who could drain his liver abscesses to temporarily relieve the pain and stop the sepsis. Bruce set a goal to live until November 11 to reach his fiftieth birthday, which he did.

In early December, he awoke one morning with fever and chills and was so prostrate that he could not sit up or get out of bed. His doctor came to the house and gave him intravenous steroids to block the effects of the sepsis and keep him alive even though the doctor knew that the survival was only temporary. This was the same doctor who had given him the extra allergy shots and precipitated his pulmonary problems several years earlier.

When Dad learned of this, he wondered why the doctor had not let Bruce die quickly from his incurable cancer rather than save him for a slow painful death. I wondered the same thing.

Bruce spent several weeks in the hospital. Because of the politics of the Stanford Hospital, or perhaps the financial situation of the private radiology group, he could not have radiation in the hospital. He had to be sent by ambulance to the radiology group's private facility for each treatment. Many days he did not feel well enough for the gurney transfers and ambulance ride so he refused treatment. People with liver disease often lose their appetite. He would not eat so the doctors approached Judy about putting in a feeding tube to keep him alive for a few added weeks.

Dad called Judy to tell her that he wanted to come to California to see Bruce before he died. She told him that he would only be in the way and complicate matters if he came. Judy told him that she would not meet him at the airport and that he would have to stay in a motel and rent a car and be completely on his own. He did not feel up to this so he stayed in Arizona, but was very unhappy at not being able to see Bruce.

Letha and I went to see Bruce during our Christmas break. We offered to meet Dad there to help him, but Dad declined. He told me that he thought Judy would keep him from spending much time with Bruce.

Bruce was in the hospital and not feeling well. When we took Judy to dinner to give her a break, she asked me about the feeding tube. I explained to her that Bruce was dying and taking pain medication as often as they would let him. His affairs were in order and he was going to die soon, but he would not return to any quality of life by being fed so prolonging his life for a painful death would not do him any favor. The only ones to benefit by keeping him alive longer were the doctors who would continue to have billable days until he died.

When Judy refused the feeding tube, the doctors sent him home to die. Judy had a hospital bed put in the living room near the first-floor bathroom. She was given a supply of Demerol to give him for pain. The doctor would not prescribe morphine, which most doctors agree is much better for cancer pain, because "Bruce might become addicted to it before he died." This is the exact antithesis to hospice care. Dad told me that he thought the denial of morphine was absurd and incompetent.

Bruce died the third week of January 1987. Letha and I went to California for the funeral, but left Scott in school in Galveston with friends looking after him. We offered to look after Dad if he came, but he was bitter about being denied the chance to see Bruce before he died and refused to come. He said that seeing him dead would not replace being able to see him and talk with him before he died.

I tried to establish a memorial in Bruce's name at Middlebury College in Vermont. Bruce had spent a year in Madrid studying and received a master's degree in Spanish literature from Middlebury. My son, Scott, went to Middlebury and majored in Italian and art history. He spent his junior year in Florence, Italy, at the Middlebury outpost there. Scott told me that the computers at the Florentine school were antiquated and barely operational. I decided to donate money to the Middlebury language department to replace the computers in Italy and name the computer room after Bruce.

I contacted the Middlebury development office and made the offer to them. They replied that I should just donate to the general fund that helped pay scholarships. When I replied that I wanted something specific that would bear Bruce's name, they replied that his name would be listed with other donors on a contribution list. They would not accept my offer. Their loss!

Chapter 35

After Mom died, we would go to Mesa during spring break each year to help Dad prepare his income taxes and have a visit with him. In 1986, Letha had an important meeting in Texas, so Scott went with me to Phoenix. Scott's job was to keep Dad occupied while I did the taxes. Otherwise, Dad would hover over me and ask questions about everything. Mom had always done the tax returns, so he did not understand what was taxed and what was not. Dad's income was from his brokerage account, and he did not have many deductions since he owned their house without a mortgage.

Scott was in high school by then. He had several long conversations with Dad, which led Dad to change his opinion about Scott. He always thought that Scott was a spoiled child with whom he had little in common. Dad told Scott many of his stories, and Scott asked the right questions. Dad decided that there was hope for Scott.

When I was not doing the taxes, Dad brought me books and medical instruments that he wanted me to have. He got out Sheriff Rader's pistol and a small bag of bullets from the top drawer of his dresser and gave it to me. He told me the story of the car thieves in Normal again.

After Bruce died in 1987, I went to Mesa to visit Dad. He told me that Judy was pestering him about his will. When Mom died, Bruce advised him to put his house into tenants in common ownership with Bruce and me. Bruce had insisted that both wives sign waivers to exclude them from any interest in his house in case one of us died or was divorced. Letha had objected, but Judy insisted that they should do as Bruce wished. Both wives had signed the waivers.

Dad put the house in common tenancy with right of survival, meaning that the title was in Dad's, Bruce's, and my name and, if someone died, the survivors would have joint ownership regardless of who died so there would be no inheritance tax on the house.

Now that Bruce had died, Judy wanted back in for half of the house and inclusion in Dad's estate. Dad was still very unhappy with her for denying his chance to see Bruce before he died and did not want to accede to Judy's requests.

Dad told me that he was reluctant to agree to this because he did not want Judy's next husband to spend the money he had worked for so hard. My grandfather Bentzen had set up trusts for Mom and her brother, Roy, but limited the income from the trust to Roy's wife if Roy died. The trust would eliminate all payment if she remarried. Dad considered a similar trust, but I convinced him to keep it simple and not worry about what happened after he was gone.

He immediately contacted his lawyer and made the changes in his will to treat Judy and me equally with the estate trusts. This change put Judy back in the will. (Judy has not remarried since Bruce's death.)

He also wanted to leave something to his only grandson whom he had decided was a nice young man. I convinced him to set up generation-skipping trust funds from the estate for Judy and for me with Scott as survivor and to leave the house title as it was for me to sell and use for Scott's college education. Dad decided that arrangement would satisfy his wishes. I thought this arrangement would also remove the problem and hard feelings about the way the house was handled.

Dad knew I was coming to help him with his taxes in April of 1987 so he had been delaying another TUR for his prostate. I learned when I arrived in Arizona that he had catheterized himself to delay the surgery. He scheduled the surgery for the time I would be there. He was to go into the hospital on Monday morning, so I had arranged to stay for the surgery.

The day before surgery, Dad called me out to the patio to talk. I think he thought he was going to die soon because he told me about a letter that Mom had written to him years ago. He produced a leather folder and removed the letter from it. He told me that he had kept the letter in his dresser all these years and wanted me to have it now.

In the letter, Mom had told him that Richard, the man for whom she had left Dad, had not turned out to be the love of her life. She realized that she still loved Dad very much, and she wanted him to take her back. He had apparently told her in another letter that he was so busy and so committed to his patients that he could never marry. In Mom's letter, she pleaded that she could make his life better by looking after him while he pursued his devotion to his patients. She promised that she would never complain about his long hours and his concern for his patients if it seemed more than for her.

He told me that he was still upset about having given half of his money to Mom to protect it from lawsuits that had never occurred while Mom never divided her inheritance with him. After her inheritance, Mom always had more money than Dad, and sometimes she reminded him of that when she wanted to spend money. He mentioned that Mom always handled the home checkbook. Since she sometimes did the bookkeeping for the office, she also had control of the practice checkbook, but he never thought she overspent and never begrudged her anything that she bought. He came from a very poor background and had lived simply, except for his travel.

Dad told me that he was aware that Bruce and I were concerned by their constant arguing, but he wanted me to know that he had always loved Mom and had taken care of her as best as he knew how. He had tried to give her everything she wanted, and he thought she had enjoyed a good life. He was glad that he had outlived her so that she did not have to care for him or to live alone after he died.

We had a nice dinner at home on Sunday night, the night before his surgery, and watched television in the family room that evening. Dad told me that he was feeling abdominal distention and asked me to get his stethoscope from his dresser. He had me listen to his abdomen and then listened to it himself. He did not have bowel sounds, which meant that he was getting an ileus. (His bowels had stopped functioning and were filling with gas.)

I called his urologist to tell him since the urologic surgery was scheduled for the next day. I was referred to his partner by the answering service. The partner called back after about an hour, so I told him the problem. He asked me why I had called him rather than Dad's internist. He did not want to deal with the situation. He told me to just take Dad to the emergency room and hung up.

We went to the emergency room and checked in. Dad's abdomen was so distended that he could not sit in the straight chairs in the waiting room so he lay on the floor. I snuck into the emergency room and returned with a gurney for him to lie on. After about a half hour, they took him into the treatment area. They hooked him to a monitor, and the medical doctor on call examined him and decided that his problem was probably a bowel obstruction so she called a surgeon.

When the surgeon arrived and examined Dad, he decided that Dad did not have an obstruction and called the internist back. The internist then told me that dad probably had impacted bowels like so many old men so they would admit him to the hospital and would give him enemas for treatment.

I knew that Dad had not been constipated so the diagnosis of impaction was improbable, but I decided not to become Dad's doctor but let his doctor handle the situation.

Once he was in his hospital room, about midnight, I went home to get some sleep so I could come back early in the morning. When I arrived in the morning, he was still distended and very uncomfortable. He had not received an enema, and the catheter that he had placed by himself several days before was connected to a collecting bag that was empty. I asked the nurse when the bag had been emptied, so she went to the nurse's station to check his chart. She returned to tell me that it had been connected at midnight and had never been emptied.

I pointed out to the nurse that he had not put out any urine since admission so his urinary tract must be obstructed. She left to call his doctor with this news. She returned with a syringe and gave him a shot in the arm. I reminded the nurse that I was a doctor and asked what she had given him. She said it was Lasix, a potent diuretic, to drive his kidneys. I thought that giving an obstructed patient a diuretic was contraindicated because it would increase the pressure in the obstructed system and might rupture his obstructed ureters or kidneys, giving him peritonitis.

In about twenty minutes, he suddenly put out about a liter of urine. The pressure from the Lasix had blown his obstruction open at least partially. Shortly after that, they sent him for an abdominal CT scan that determined that both of his ureters were blocked and dilated to several times normal size.

His urology doctor's partner came that afternoon to tell us that the cancer had probably spread to block the ureters where they entered his bladder just above the prostate. They would have to do a cystoscopic exam and put stents in the ureters to keep them open. They did not want to operate until things had quieted down and his ileus had subsided. They would wait a week or more before placing the stents and hope that he did not obstruct again before then.

The partner of his regular internist came in at about 7:00 p.m. and told Dad that they would start enemas to treat his ileus. Dad questioned this, but the internist was still working on the theory that he was a typical old man who had been constipated and become impacted although Dad's history did not support the conclusion.

I asked the internist to step out into the hall so I could talk with him. I wanted to know why they had not put in a nasogastric tube to treat the ileus. He looked at me blankly and asked why he should do that. I told him that every surgeon knew that a nasogastric tube was the best way to treat an ileus. I guessed that since he was an internist, he was not used to treating postoperative ileus.

He thought about it for a minute and replied that Dad was a doctor so we should ask him what he thought about a tube. When the doctor asked Dad if it would be all right to put a tube into his stomach if the ileus was still there in the morning, Dad looked up at him and said, "What in the hell are you waiting for? That is the only way to treat an ileus." The doctor immediately ordered and N-G tube, and a nurse came in to put it down. Dad was comfortable in about twenty minutes with noticeable decrease in his distention.

(I learned a lot about ileus when I was an intern and again when I was a resident in ophthalmology. During my three years of ophthalmology residency, I was called to see three different patients who had undergone abdominal exploratory surgery for bowel obstruction and ileus but no obstruction was found.

An eye consult was requested after the surgery when the patient was noted to have a red eye. These patients all had angle-closure glaucoma attacks that caused them to develop ileus. Their intraocular pressures were all elevated, and the angle between the cornea and the iris in the involved eye was still closed. Treating the glaucoma resolved their problem.)

(For some reason, the body reacts to obstruction of a hollow organ by shutting down the gastrointestinal system. This is known as the "obstructed hollow viscus syndrome." Hollow organs include large or small bowel, appendix, gallbladder or bile ducts, urinary bladder, ureters, kidney, and the eyeball. In my father's case, it was his ureters that were obstructed, causing his ileus.)

(Dr. Carl Moyer, the chief of surgery at Washington University, taught us that rectal tubes or enemas would not deflate an ileus, but a nasogastric tube, through the nose and the esophagus into the stomach, would immediately relieve the abdominal distention. During the surgical rotations of my internship, we always put down a nasogastric tube at the end of abdominal surgical cases to prevent the usual ileus after surgery. It usually takes two to four days for the intestines to begin to work after abdominal surgery.)

By Tuesday morning, Dad was feeling better. The urologist had told him that they would probably wait two weeks to place the stents unless he obstructed again. I decided to go home to Texas and return in time for the stent surgery. I asked the nurse to call me in Galveston if there was any change and left a note on his chart with my home and office phone numbers.

The next weekend, on Easter morning, I was awakened at about 6:00 a.m. by a telephone call from one of Dad's lapidary friends. The hospital had called him and told him to come to the hospital because Dad had taken a "turn for the worse." These friends called me to see if I knew what had happened.

I had made a note of the phone number in the nurse's station, so I called and asked for the nurse. They could not find her before I was cut off. I called back a few minutes later and got the nurse right away. I asked about my dad, and she told me that he had "taken a turn for the worse." I reminded her that I was a doctor and asked for more details. She told me that when she had checked him about a half hour before, "he had no vital signs." That told me that he was dead.

I asked her what was being done, and she immediately became defensive and reminded me that he had passed out copies of his living will when he entered the hospital to anyone who would take one. It requested not to resuscitate him. The nurse told me that they were waiting for the doctor from the emergency room to come to the floor to pronounce him dead. I asked her to have his doctor call me when it was convenient.

It was Easter Sunday and Letha was to read the scripture in church, so we went to church. At about three o'clock that afternoon (2:00 p.m. Arizona time), the doctor called. He told me that "he was sorry to hear about my father." He had heard that "he died in his sleep."

I remembered Dad's telling my grandfather years ago that he thought that dying in one's sleep was "a good way to go." My grandfather's quick reply was, "How do you know? You've never done it."

I told the doctor that I wanted a postmortem exam performed on Dad. The doctor replied that he died in the hospital so a post was not necessary. I explained that Dad was the oldest patient on whom Dr. Cooley had done CABG surgery at that date, so I wanted the report for Dr. Cooley at Methodist Hospital in Houston. It would be important for Dr. Cooley's research for him to know the state of Dad's coronary bypasses this long after the surgery.

I also told his doctor that Dad's biopsies had always been reported as adenocarcinoma of undetermined origin. I wanted an opinion from the pathologist about the source of the cancer. Dad had smoked almost all his adult life and was therefore susceptible to bladder cancer. I wanted to know, for my own future planning, what kind of cancer to watch for as I aged.

The doctor told me that the pathologists would not do autopsies anymore because they were afraid of AIDS. I asked the doctor if he had any reason to believe that Dad had AIDS. He replied, "Of course not." I told the doctor to have the pathologist call me if he had any objections.

The doctor then told me that Medicare would not pay for the ambulance to take him to the funeral home after the autopsy once they used an ambulance to transport the body to the pathologist's laboratory. I told him to send me the bill for the ambulance. I assured him that I was not planning to sue him over the results of the autopsy.

I had seen the monitor in the emergency room and was surprised by how good Dad's EKG looked thirteen years after quadruple coronary artery bypass surgery. In the ER, because of his distress, he had a tachycardia of 120 beats per minute, but no ST segment changes or abnormal T waves to indicate cardiac problems. His heart was working very well in the ER.

I concluded that when he died, his electrolytes were out of balance because of his ileus, the urinary obstruction, the diuretics they gave him, and the intravenous fluids he had been given while his ileus resolved. The electrolyte imbalance had probably caused a cardiac arrhythmia that led to his death. The other possibility was a sudden stroke.

As I took Dad to the hospital, he had pointed out the nursing home he wanted to go to if they did not let him go home from the hospital. When I pooh-poohed that, he told me that he thought the end was near. He had been feeling very weak for about a month and knew something was wrong.

I thought that the doctor's "hearing about my father's death" was indicative of his involvement in the case. I never saw him at the hospital or talked with him on the phone. I never talked directly or on the phone with his urologist either.

I never received a bill for the ambulance or a copy of the autopsy. I doubt that Dr. Cooley received one either. By the time I realized this, it was too late. Dad had requested to be cremated with his ashes scattered on Red Mountain, next to Mom. There was no way to go back and do the autopsy. I hoped that the poor quality of medical care my father received is not indicative of the general level of care received by Medicare patients in the Mesa area, but reports I have heard were not encouraging.

It was ironic that my dad, who had showed such clinical competency coupled with concern and compassion for his patients, would receive such incompetent and impassive care as he died. The Hippocratic Oath requires that doctors care for everyone, but especially other physicians, with care and compassion to the utmost of their ability. I was glad that he died quietly in his sleep, possibly without pain, on Easter morning before his cancer became painful and completely drained him of his strength.

We had a memorial service at the same church where Mom's service was held. The funeral home made arrangements for a small plane to drop Dad's ashes on Red Mountain. Lee Long officiated again at the same picnic area on the Verde River. We prayed and watched the ashes settle on the mountain at sunrise on the day after the memorial service.

Breaking up the house was going to take some work. It was filled with the souvenirs of his travels all over the world and the many cherished memories of his career. Dad had paid off the rental furniture, enabling us to sell the house furnished. Scott was seventeen then, and Dad told me that Scott should have his car if he did not come back home from the hospital. It was a tan Pontiac sedan that did not appeal to Scott, so I sold it and gave the money to Scott to buy a used car of his choice.

It was April, so we decided to wait until school was out to come back to Arizona to close the house and put it on the market. I talked with Dad's lawyer who assured me that everything was in order. He could take care of the will and inheritance taxes until I came back to close the house.

POSTLUDE

AFTER DAD DIED, I BEGAN thinking of a fitting memorial for him. He had made his mark in Normal, Illinois, and was best known by people there. He had a long loyalty and fondness for Brokaw Hospital. Most of his surgery was done there, and he played a leadership role in the governance of the hospital. He would always roll out of bed and drive the three blocks to the hospital whenever called, regardless of who was the designated doctor on call.

The event that was most prominent in the stories he told about Brokaw Hospital was the time he gave the first citrated blood transfusion to be done in Bloomington–Normal. His other blood-related story was using a Turkel pneumothorax needle to give a badly burned child a blood transfusion, directly into the marrow cavity of the sternum. It saved the child's life when extensive burns and shock made it impossible to find a vein for the transfusion. I decided to find out how the blood bank at the hospital was functioning.

In the years after Dad retired, Brokaw Hospital had merged with Mennonite Hospital in Bloomington when hospitals were having trouble surviving. Brokaw was twice the size it had been when Dad practiced there, but it was still at the same location. The blood bank for both hospitals was at Brokaw.

I contacted the administration. They told me that much of the equipment in the blood bank was aging and should be replaced. The administrator was new, but he had heard of my father and was amenable to dedicating the blood bank to Dad. When I told him about the first citrated blood transfusion, he became enthusiastic about the dedication. I gave them the money to buy several pieces of processing equipment for the needed replacements and a new blood refrigerator.

The hospital insisted that Letha, Scott, and I come from Texas for the dedication. Judy came from California, and about twenty of Dad's surviving friends attended the dedication. The hospital had a bronze plaque made with a bas relief of Dad's face and the inscription, "Harry C. Barber, MD Blood Bank." The plaque is placed next to the door to the blood bank.

I have not been back to Normal for years, but I am sure that the plaque is still there. It is a small memorial to a man who dedicated himself to treating disease and helping his fellowman. He was a boy who grew up on a small farm on a bluff overlooking the Missouri River near Kansas City. He was very intelligent and creative and applied these characteristics with tremendous drive to reach his goal of becoming a doctor like his uncle. As a doctor, he continued to invent and create new treatments for the ethical and moral care of his beloved patients.

CPSIA information can be obtained
at www.ICGtesting.com
Printed in the USA
BVHW030242200820
586887BV00002B/2/J